THE MESCHINO

OPTIMAL LIVING PROGRAM

THE MESCHINO
OPTIMAL LIVING PROGRAM

SEVEN STEPS TO A HEALTHY, FIT, AGE-RESISTANT BODY

Dr. James Meschino

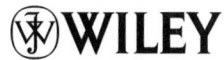

John Wiley & Sons Canada, Ltd.

National Library of Canada Cataloguing in Publication Data

Meschino, James, 1954-
    The Meschino optimal living program : seven steps to a
    healthy, fit, age-resistant body / James Meschino.

ISBN 0-470-83487-0

1. Health.　2. Nutrition.　3. Physical fitness.　I. Title.
RA776.M475 2004　　613'.0434　　C2004-906044-9

Production Credits:

Cover design: Adrian So R.G.D.
Interior text design: Pat Loi & Adrian So R.G.D.
Front cover photo: Karen Whylie/Coyote Photos
Printer: Transcontinental Printing

John Wiley & Sons Canada, Ltd
6045 Freemont Blvd.
Mississauga, ON
L5R 4J3
www.wiley.ca

Printed in Canada
10 9 8 7 6 5 4 3 2 1

Contents

Acknowledgments

I would like to acknowledge Don Loney, who, after reviewing other books and educational materials I have developed, suggested that I write this book, and who recommended it for publication to his co-workers at John Wiley & Sons Canada.

Don, I am most grateful to you for encouraging me to write this book and for affording me the opportunity to share my program with so many people. I also wish to acknowledge my editor Jan Walter who did a magnificent job of smoothing out my writing, translating complex scientific concepts into understandable language, and keeping each part of the message contained in this book on target and accurate. Jan, I could not have done this without your help, and I am grateful for the interest you showed in the subject matter and your relentless attention to detail.

I would also like to acknowledge the editing support of Elizabeth McCurdy, project manager, and Martha Wilson, copyeditor, who did an outstanding and meticulous job of fine tuning the manuscript and layout of the book. And to the other individuals at John Wiley & Sons Canada who contributed to the making of this book and its promotion. I am most grateful for all of your efforts.

Finally, I wish to thank all of the researchers whose studies I quote and reference throughout the *Meschino Optimal Living Program*. It is your work that has shown us that attention to diet, supplementation and exercise, can slow the aging process, reduce risk of degenerative diseases and greatly enhance our quality of life.

Introduction

Welcome to *The Meschino Optimal Living Program.* The system described in these pages is the culmination of 25 years of personal research and clinical experience. Its purpose is to provide you with a proven, life-long strategy for maintaining your ideal weight, enhancing your fitness and energy levels, improving your cardio-vascular health, and reducing your risk of degenerative and age-related diseases. Easy to follow and highly effective, this nutrition, exercise and supplementation program equips you with both the knowledge and the plan of action to achieve the healthy, well-functioning body that nature intended.

Modern research has long established that proper eating habits, regular exercise, and the right nutritional supplements can slow or reverse many aspects of the aging process. The benefits are legion: the maintenance of immune function, bone density, cognitive ability, and sexual virility; a radiant appearance, increased energy, and a sense of well-being; the prevention or postponement of the most common diseases that plague the western world; a longer, more productive and rewarding life.

I wrote this book with one truth in mind: the simple daily effort required to optimize the health of your body is well within your ability, your means, and your timetable. And isn't good health worth that effort? If you become sick or disabled, the goals you have set for yourself will almost certainly become more difficult to achieve and the social, recreational and athletic activities you enjoy less pleasurable, perhaps even impossible.

For more than two decades, I have taught the principles of this program to healthcare professionals throughout Canada and the United States and have incorporated them into wellness initiatives for numerous corporations. I have seen excellent clinical results among the patients treated in my own nutritional consulting practice. Unfortunately, many North Americans either do not realize the benefits of this combined approach to nutrition, exercise and supplementation, or they are willing to live with the consequences of ignoring the basic laws of healthy living.

We are currently experiencing an epidemic of degenerative diseases, many of which are preventable or can be greatly reduced in severity, according to top experts from around the world. For example, data published in the Journal of the National Cancer Institute in 1996 by Dr. Walter Willet of Harvard University indicated that between 70 and 90% of all cancers could be avoided through more prudent dietary and lifestyle behaviors. It is well accepted within the medical community that vascular disease leading to heart attack and stroke, the leading killers in our society, is primarily caused by poor eating and lifestyle habits. The same is true for the alarming increases in the incidence of Type 2 diabetes and osteoporosis. Furthermore, there is evidence that deficiencies of certain nutrients are behind many cases of cataracts and macular degeneration of the eye, as well the development of age-related dementia and cognitive decline.

These facts illustrate that in the majority of cases, the serious health afflictions we fear are not the fault of our genes but rather the way we choose to live our lives. And that means there is something you can do about it: choose the right foods, commit to the right exercise program and add the right supplements to your diet, and you will significantly reduce your risk of these afflictions and dramatically slow the effects of aging.

In the pages that follow, I'll introduce you to the Two Staple Nutrition System, a plan that ensures that you'll eat the foods your body needs to be healthy, lean and disease-resistant. I'll show you how to incorporate an appropriate and personalized exercise program into your life. Plus, I'll explain precisely what nutritional supplement combinations you should take every day and at every stage of your life to counter aging and protect against disease. Scientists tell us that with proper attention to diet, exercise, specific supplements and other lifestyle measures, we have the potential to live at least 120 years and to enjoy a high quality of life throughout this lifespan. *The Meschino Optimal Living Program* explains the science on which these statements are based and shows you how to translate science and clinical knowledge into a practical, daily program that is accessible and available to everyone who truly cares about their health and wellness.

STEP I

Build Your Nutrition Foundation

The first step in building a lifestyle program for a healthy, fit, age-resistant body is to understand how various nutrients work in your body. Nutrients can either promote your health and prevent disease, or detract from your health and encourage the development of degenerative diseases leading to premature death. Understand how various nutrients affect your health, and you can visualize what happens inside your body every time you consume carbohydrate foods, high-protein foods, saturated fat, cholesterol, omega-3 fats, monounsaturated fats, and other nutrients. *So* let's spend some time examining how your body processes the foods you eat.

Carbohydrates

Thanks to the recent high-protein, low-carbohydrate diet craze, there is a great deal of confusion about carbohydrate foods. Do they promote health, delay aging, and prevent disease? What is their role in weight loss?

The first thing to appreciate is that many carbohydrate foods are provided to us by the good earth: fruits and vegetables; grains (such as rice); cereal products (for example, wheat); and legumes, including beans and peas. Naturally-occurring carbohydrates can be manipulated by food processing to make the modified carbohydrates that are found in breads, breakfast cereals, pasta, crackers, jams and jellies, and sugar. Although the different carbohydrates we consume vary in terms of their health-promoting features, all carbohydrate foods, including white sugar, have one thing in common: they all provide the building blocks from which your body makes glucose. Glucose is the simple sugar molecule that serves as an essential energy source for virtually every cell in the body. If your blood sugar level drops, meaning the level of glucose in the blood is abnormally low, then the cells can no longer function at their best. This is why you are likely to feel shaky, light-headed, irritable, and unable to concentrate, if you go past your usual mealtime without eating. These symptoms are a direct result of low blood glucose levels.

Your body digests carbohydrate foods and produces glucose for energy in a highly efficient way. After ingestion, your digestive enzymes go to work to release the individual sugars in these foods, allowing them to pass into the bloodstream. Once in the blood-stream, carbohydrate sugars travel to the liver where they are converted into glucose by the action of specific liver enzymes. The glucose is returned to the bloodstream, where it becomes a continuous source of energy for the body's cells. It doesn't matter if you eat a potato, a bowl of rice, a plate of pasta, a piece of fruit, or a salad—the carbohydrates in these foods will all be converted into glucose, which will help power most of the body's cells. Some of the glucose will be used immediately and some stored in the liver for future use. Between meals, the liver releases this stored glucose, called glycogen, to the bloodstream to meet the energy demands of your body.

If you fail to consume adequate amounts of carbohydrate foods and deprive your cells of energy, you may develop the condi-tion known as hypoglycemia, which means "low blood sugar." Hypoglycemia affects the brain and nervous system quite dramati-cally, because brain cells and other nerves rely on glucose for up to 95 percent of their energy needs. As described earlier, the symptoms of hypoglycemia include fatigue, irritability, nervousness, a dull headache, and so forth. Thus it is imperative to maintain blood glucose levels by consuming the right amount of carbohydrates each day.

Of course some carbohydrate foods are better for you than others. Not only do they provide carbohydrate energy, they may also contain protective nutrients that help defend us against cancer and heart disease. Remember that some carbohydrate foods release their sugars faster than others and are therefore absorbed more rapidly into the bloodstream. Carbohydrate foods that are absorbed too quickly are more likely to be converted into fat and triglycerides within the body and can also produce a sugar rush, from too sudden a rise in blood sugar. This can result in weight gain, a rebound drop in blood sugar (hypoglycemia) or an increase in the risk of developing diabetes. Athletes may want to consume carbohydrates that are absorbed quickly into the bloodstream, as doing so can enhance performance in many endurance events. But day to day, most of your carbohydrates should come from carbohydrate foods that are absorbed more slowly from the intestinal tract and that contain the protective nutrients that reduce the risk of cancer, heart disease, and other degenerative diseases.

The Right Amount and Right Type of Carbohydrate Foods

Your body requires sufficient carbohydrate energy each day to sustain its peak functional state, but that's not to say that you can eat unlimited carbohydrate calories without consequences. Overconsuming carbohydrate calories will increase your body fat and your blood triglyceride levels, those fats found in the blood that are associated with heart disease risk. However, avoiding carbohydrate foods is an equally critical mistake that many carbohydrate-phobic dieters are making these days. The key is to consume the right amount and right type of carbohydrate foods, appropriate to your lifestyle and activity level. Used wisely, carbohydrate foods will elevate your energy level, boost your defenses against disease, help you attain and maintain your ideal body weight without feeling deprived, and improve your performance in most exercise and athletic endeavors. Depending on your level of physical activity, carbohydrate foods should make up 45 to 65 percent of your total calories. The more active you are, the greater the requirement for carbohydrate consumption. If you are more sedentary, then you cannot consume the same quantity or percentage of carbohydrate calories as a highly active person without experiencing weight gain and other health problems.

Over the years nutritionists and dieticians have told us that there are two types of carbohydrates to be aware of: complex carbohydrates and simple carbohydrates, sometimes referred to as low-glycemic and high-glycemic carbohydrate foods, respectively. Yet this approach to carbohydrate identification does not tell the whole story. If you are truly interested in living as long as possible in a healthy, fit, age-resistant body, then you have to understand carbohydrate foods on a more sophisticated level.

I have broken down carbohydrate foods into five categories in order for you to fully understand how carbohydrate choices impact your health. Some categories should be emphasized more than others, but all five have their place in human nutrition and optimal wellness. In order of their beneficial importance to a healthy diet, they are:

Category 1 – Low-Glycemic, Nutrient-Dense Carbohydrates

Category 2 – High-Glycemic, Nutrient-Dense Carbohydrates

Category 3 – High-Fiber Grains and Starchy Carbohydrates

Category 4 – Low-Fiber Grains and Starchy Carbohydrates

Category 5 – Refined Sugars

Category 1 — Low-Glycemic, Nutrient-Dense Carbohydrates

These carbohydrate foods:

- slowly release their carbohydrates into the bloodstream from the intestinal tract;
- are low in total calories and do not readily encourage weight gain or blood sugar imbalances;
- are a rich source of vitamins, minerals and other protective nutrients, known as phytonutrients, which help reduce the risk of cancer, heart disease, and other degenerative diseases.

Category 1 carbohydrates are extremely beneficial to the body, and should be a main focus of your daily carbohydrate intake. The choices include asparagus, spinach, broccoli, cauliflower, Brussels sprouts, cabbage, bok choy, rapini, collard greens, turnips, tomatoes,peppers, onions, cantaloupe, granny smith apples, radicchio, romaine lettuce, beans, peas, and lentils. Many of these contain powerful protective nutrients. Try to consume at least three servings of the following carbohydrate foods each day.

Cruciferous Vegetables (broccoli, Brussels sprouts, cabbage, cauliflower, bok choy, turnips)—individuals with high intakes of these vegetables throughout their lifetimes show a significant reduction in the incidence of colon cancer, breast cancer, and prostate cancer. These vegetables contain indole-3-carbinol, which enhances the ability of our detoxification enzymes to neutralize and remove carcinogens from the bloodstream and the cells. Indole-3-carbinol also promotes the conversion of estrone, one of the body's estrogen hormones, into 2-hydroxy-estrone—instead of the potentially harmful 16-hydroxy-estrone, which is associated with an increased risk of breast cancer. Indole-3-carbinol may block the synthesis of estrone hormone in fat cells, which is associated with a reduction in risk of breast and prostate cancer. I suggest that you eat cruciferous vegetables every day.

Tomatoes—tomatoes are a rich source of the antioxidant lycopene. Higher intakes of lycopene have been linked to significant reductions in prostate cancer and cervical cancer. Lycopene is a sister compound to beta-carotene and is one of many carotenoids found in fruits and vegetables. It gives tomatoes their red color and red grapefruit its pink tinge. Two extensive U.S. studies, the Health Professionals Follow-Up Study and the Physicians' Health Study, suggest that higher intakes of lycopene, mostly from tomatoes and tomato products (such as pasta sauces) and higher blood levels of lycopene were linked to a lower risk of prostate cancer. Lycopene has been shown to concentrate in the male prostate gland, where it provides antioxidant protection against free radicals—aggressive compounds that randomly attack body tissues—and exhibits other anti-cancer effects. These effects of lycopene are similarily important in the prevention of cervical cancer in women. Lycopene is a fat-soluble nutrient and therefore must be consumed with a bit of fat in order to be absorbed into the bloodstream. Use olive oil in your pasta sauce. Or eat salads that are dressed with olive oil-based dressings. (Drinking tomato juice on an empty stomach or eating tomatoes with no concomitant fat consumption means no lycopene will be absorbed from the intestinal tract into the bloodstream.) A daily serving of tomatoes or tomato-based products is highly recommended.

Spinach, Asparagus and Other Dark Green Leafy Vegetables—these vegetables contain lutein and zeaxanthin, two carotenoids that help prevent macular degeneration, the leading cause of blindness in individuals over the age of 55 in the United States and Canada. Lutein and zeaxanthin concentrate in the back of the eye, near the optic nerve, protecting it against damage by free radicals induced by sunlight. Studies show that a higher lifetime intake of lutein and zeaxanthin lowers the risk of macular degeneration and cataracts, and that lutein and zeaxanthin supplements can help slow the progression of macular degeneration, especially when taken along with other antioxidant supplements like vitamin C, vitamin E, selenium, and zinc.

Mostly dark green vegetables also contain beta-carotene and folic acid. Beta-carotene is an important antioxidant that may help reduce cancer risk, and folic acid is required for normal DNA synthesis in every cell in the body. Many individuals in North America who do not take a daily multivitamin and mineral supplement suffer marginal deficiency in folic acid; that makes them more prone to certain colon and breast cancers. In women of childbearing age, there is increased risk of giving birth to children with spinal birth defects, such as spina bifida. Consuming dark green leafy vegetables—not iceberg lettuce—should also be part of your daily carbohydrate intake strategy.

Beans, Peas and Lentils—these legumes contain lignans and plant-based sterols, which provide many disease-prevention benefits to the body. Lignans help block the overproduction of estrone hormone in fat cells, which in turn is associated with a reduced incidence of breast and prostate cancer. Plant-based sterols, such as beta-sitosterol, are known to block the conversion of testosterone into dihydrotestosterone, an effect that has been linked to the prevention of prostate enlargement and prostate cancer. Plant sterols have also been demonstrated to block the replication of certain breast cancer cells, improve immune function, and help keep blood cholesterol in a safe range by preventing the absorption of cholesterol and bile acids from the intestinal tract into the bloodstream. Furthermore, beans, peas, and lentils contain the kind of fiber that improves bowel function (thereby reducing the risk of colon cancer) and that lowers blood cholesterol (thus helping prevent heart attack and stroke).

Soybeans and related soy products, like tofu, miso soup, and soy nuts, contain isoflavones, which are strongly associated with a reduced risk of breast and prostate cancer. Since many soy products are high enough in protein to be classified as protein foods, we will examine them at greater length in the protein section of this chapter.

Onions and Garlic—onions and garlic, allium-containing vegetables, have a specialized group of disulfide compounds that exhibit potent anti-cancer, anti-heart disease, and immune-stimulating properties.

Category 2—High-Glycemic, Nutrient-Dense Carbohydrates

These carbohydrates:

- contain a lot of simple sugars that are absorbed quickly into the bloodstream, which can produce a sugar rush or hasten their conversion into fat, if they are consumed in excess; (This is the only negative feature of Category 2 carbohydrates.)

- are a rich source of many protective nutrients—such as carotenes, flavonoids, vitamins, and minerals—which are important in the prevention of cancer, heart disease, and other degenerative diseases;

- are a good source of cholesterol-lowering fiber.

Category 2 carbohydrates are found in all sweet-tasting fruits (oranges, clementines, nectarines, peaches, plums, grapes, pineapple, honeydew melon, watermelon, strawberries, blueberries, cranberries, kiwi, papaya, mango, dates, figs, dried fruits); fruit juices (which should always be diluted at least 50 percent with water); all sweet vegetables (squash, yams, sweet potatoes, carrots, corn, beets); and jams and jellies.

Factor at least one or two servings of these foods into your daily carbohydrate intake:

Orange-yellow fruits and vegetables—are generally high in beta-carotene and other carotenoids, such as lutein, which provide antioxidant protection to many parts of the body. Studies indicate that people with high intakes of orange-yellow fruits and vegetables and dark green leafy vegetables have a significantly lower incidence of various cancers, heart disease, cataracts, or macular degeneration of the eye. In addition, one-sixth of all the beta-carotene consumed can be converted into vitamin A by your body, if your body requires more. Vitamin A serves many important functions and has also been shown to exhibit anti-cancer properties.

Dark Blue Fruits and Vegetables—the dark blue colour of blueberries, bilberries, and blue-purple grapes is due to the presence of specific flavonoids. These flavonoid compounds provide antioxidant effects; protect the eye from ultraviolet light damage; and can strengthen the blood vessels, helping to prevent ruptures, hemorrhage, and the formation of varicose veins.

Jams, Jellies, Apples, Peaches, Pears, and Plums—these carbohydrate foods are an excellent source of cholesterol-lowering fiber, which helps prevent heart disease and stroke.

Category 3—High-Fiber Grains and Starchy Carbohydrates

These carbohydrates:

- contain a lot of carbohydrate calories per serving. Unless you are exercising regularly at a high level of intensity, over consumption of Category 3 carbohydrates will hasten their conversion to fat and lead to a rise in body fat and triglyceride levels. People who work out regularly and are engaged in en-durance activities should consume more of these carbohydrates to help replenish their carbohydrate stores on daily basis;

- These kinds of carbohydrates are a very good source of the type of dietary fiber that is associated with reduced risk of colon cancer and improved function of the large bowel. A small daily dosage of Category 3 carbohydrates can provide significant health benefits to the bowels.

Category 3 carbohydrate foods include brown rice, couscous, high-fiber/low-fat breakfast cereals, whole wheat and whole grain breads, high-fiber/low-fat crackers and biscuits, and whole wheat pasta and noodles. A low fat/high fiber breakfast cereal is one that contains at least 8 grams of fiber and no more than 1.5 grams of fat per serving (usual serving size is ⅓ or ½ cup, sometimes indicated as 28 grams or 36 grams respectively). A low fat/fiber cracker contains approximately 2.4 grams of fat and 1.5 grams of fiber per ½ ounce serving, and a high fiber bread contains 0.8-1.0 grams of fat per slice (regular slice) and 1.4-1.7 grams of fiber. (These are the criteria readers should use as a guideline when they look at nutrition labels on these products).

Category 4—Low-Fiber Grains and Starchy Carbohydrates

These carbohydrates:

- like Category 3 carbohydrates, contain many carbohydrate calories per serving. In most people, overconsumption will increase body fat and triglyceride levels;
- do not contain much fiber—and so, unlike their Category 3 counterparts, do not offer health benefits to the large bowel. However, don't think that you can never again

enjoy white bread without causing harm to your body. This simply is not the case. Just do not make it a heavy part of your daily diet.

Category 4 carbohydrates are found in white rice, white pasta, white bread, white potatoes, and low-fiber crackers made from white flour.

Category 5 — Refined Sugars

These carbohydrates:

- contain simple sugars that are rapidly absorbed into the bloodstream and can therefore upset blood glucose levels hasten the conversion of carbohydrates into fat and promote weight gain and diabetes if overconsumed;

- are essentially devoid of nutrients that protect against cancer, heart disease, and other degenerative conditions. The exception: sweet, low-fat snacks that contain some fiber ingredients.

Category 5 carbohydrate foods include white sugar, brown sugar, honey, and many refined sugar products (licorice, jujubes, hard candy, and jelly beans); low-fat frozen treats (sorbets, sherberts, low-fat frozen yogurt, and popsicles); low-fat muffins and granola bars; angel food cake.

Refined sugars are absorbed into the bloodstream extremely quickly, which can result in a rapid elevation of blood glucose levels. The pancreas must then respond by pumping large quantities of insulin into the bloodstream to lower blood sugar to normal levels. Over your lifetime, an excessive indulgence in refined sugars can over-stimulate the pancreas, forcing it to secrete more and more insulin. The insulin pushes down blood sugar levels, which can trigger a renewed craving for sweets and rebound hypoglycemia.

This recurring cycle is a common nutritional pattern, contributing to the high percentage of obese people in our society. In response to the refined sugar bombardment, the high levels of insulin secreted by the pancreas also prompt the liver to convert extra carbohydrate sugars into fat. This leads to weight gain and to elevated blood triglyceride levels, a major contributing factor to heart attacks and strokes. Weight gain produces a resistance to the effects of insulin, forcing the pancreas to secrete even higher levels in order to keep blood sugar levels from skyrocketing. A body in this condition is susceptible to the onset of adult diabetes (Type II), also known as non-insulin-dependent diabetes.

Avoid over consumption of Category 5 carbohydrates. In reasonable amounts they can be incorporated into your nutrition game plan without doing damage. (If you are exercising regularly, at a sufficient level of intensity, they pose much less of a threat.)

How Much and Which Category of Carbohydrate?

There is no doubt that your body requires the ingestion of some carbohydrate foods each day. The question is how much carbohydrate should you consume and which carbohydrates should you choose? If you are a marathon runner or participate regularly in endurance sports, then as much as 70 percent of your calories should come from carbohydrate foods. However, if you lead an essentially sedentary lifestyle, you must reduce your carbohydrate calories to as low as 45 percent of your daily caloric intake; otherwise, you will experience weight gain and a host of health problems. For health promotion, disease prevention and anti-aging, a regular exercise program must be an integral part of your lifelong game plan. Even a relatively modest regimen would allow you to consume at least 50 percent of your calories each day in the form of carbohydrates. But what proportion of your carbohydrate intake should come from each category?

Whether carbohydrate foods comprise 50, 55, or 65 percent of your daily calories, aim to select foods from the various carbohydrate categories as follows:

- **Category 1 carbohydrates** should account for approximately 40 to 45 percent of your daily carbohydrate intake.

- **Category 2 carbohydrates** should be approximately 20 to 25 percent of your daily carbohydrate intake.

- **Category 3 and Category 4 carbohydrates** should be approximately 20 to 25 percent of your daily carbohydrate intake. Emphasize Category 3 as much as possible for fiber content.

- **Category 5 carbohydrates** should be no more than 15 percent of your total daily carbohydrate intake.

Following this formula will help ensure that you consume primarily those carbohydrates that provide important protective nutrients against disease. It will help reduce the chances of weight gain and the development of Type II diabetes, while affording the freedom to consume some desserts and snacks. Be aware of the five carbohydrate categories and begin today to make smarter carbohydrate choices.

Carbohydrates and Weight Reduction

Before leaving carbohydrates behind, let's look more closely at the relationship between carbohydrates and weight loss. The popularity of high-protein/low-carbohydrate diets has persuaded many people to avoid carbohydrates. But complete abstention from carbohydrate foods has serious implications with respect to the prevention of cancer, heart disease, and other degenerative conditions. If you are overweight, don't avoid carbohydrate foods; instead, start concentrating on how to use them in conjunction with protein and a low-fat diet to lose weight. It can be easy. Over the years most of my weight loss clients have said, "I'm losing weight, and I don't even feel like I'm dieting." They are really saying that they are not experiencing the unpleasant side effects associated with carbohydrate-deprived diets—hunger, headaches, and irritability. The right amount of carbohydrate foods can help your body naturally attain and maintain your ideal weight in several ways:

- Complex carbohydrates have fewer than half the calories of the same amount of fat. One gram of a complex carbohydrate has four calories; one gram of fat has nine.

- Studies have repeatedly demonstrated that our bodies do not absorb 10 to 20 percent of the calories in many grain-based and whole wheat-based carbohydrate foods. This fact is especially true for starchy foods like pasta, bread, legumes, and rice. Our digestive enzymes cannot finish the job of breaking down these complex carbohydrate foods in the small intestines. Partially digested food passes into the large intestine; no further absorption can take place. In a sense, these are free calories. Next time you look at a calorie counter, you can subtract 10 to 20 percent of the calories listed for these items.

- Category 3 and 4 carbohydrate foods require considerable energy to digest. These energy calories are given off as heat instead of being stored as fat. The process is called thermogenesis. If you eat more of these carbohydrates than your liver can store in its glucose storage tank, 23 percent of the extra calories will be given off as heat from your body as the liver converts extra carbohydrate calories into fat. By contrast, when you eat fat, it is digested, absorbed, assimilated, transported, and stored as fat with an efficiency rate of 93 percent. The truth is that overeating carbohydrate foods, even refined sugars, is much less damaging from a weight gain perspective than eating the same number of calories of fat, especially saturated fat.

- Starchy complex carbohydrate foods such as bread, pasta, rice, and bananas make you feel full after a meal. They actually shut off the hunger message from your brain. Nutritionists call this feeling satiety—the sensation of being satisfied and content. Eliminating that feeling of hunger is an integral part of weight loss. Diets that make people feel deprived all the time are certain to fail. Fatty foods also produce that feeling of satiety, but they are much higher in calories and more damaging to your health in other ways.

- Complex carbohydrate foods provide the chemical links necessary to burn off body fat. In fact, if your carbohydrate intake is too low, you cannot completely break down body fat, and your body goes into ketosis. In this state the body begins to breakdown its muscle structure (protein) and converts it into glucose in order to prevent extreme hypoglycemia that would otherwise be life-threatening. At the same time the breakdown of fat is so rapid that some of the fat is converted to a water-soluble form called ketones, which increase the acidity of the blood. This is ketosis. This leads to the kind of weight loss that is experienced by cancer patients: up to half of the loss that occurs can be the result of your body breaking down its own muscle protein (muscles are largely made of protein) to make glucose. In this event you build up toxic wastes—ketone bodies—in your system, causing headaches, dehydration, and overwhelming hunger pangs as your blood glucose levels fluctuate at the low end of the normal range or drop below. You look sickly, emaciated, and gaunt.

This form of weight loss also slows down your metabolism. If you break down your muscle mass and convert it into glucose, then your muscles become smaller. Muscles are the motors of the body; even at rest they consume a lot of calories. The more muscle tissue you have, the faster your resting metabolic rate. Any weight loss program that encourages the breakdown of muscle tissue, rather than preserving or increasing it, will eventually slow your metabolism and raise the chances that you will regain all of the weight you lost and possibly more once you deviate from the diet—which is bound to happen if you feel carbohydrate-deprived. This is why 90-95% of individuals who lose weight from dieting gain it back within the first two years.

You must also remember that it's not necessarily just the bread and pasta that make you fat; the high-fat butter and sauces on top do much of the damage. How many overweight vegetarians have you met? Not many. Most of them are very slim, and yet their diet is comprised primarily of carbohydrates, albeit not a lot of refined sugars; they are health conscious even in regards to the carbohydrate choices they make. However, starchy carbohydrates and whole grains, fruits and vegetables from Category 1, Category 2 and Category 3 carbohydrates make up the bulk of their diet.

So it's not fair to single out carbohydrate foods in general as the main culprits driving high rates of obesity in this part of the world. The overconsumption of refined carbohydrates and, to some degree, refined grains and starches is a contributing factor, especially when combined with a sedentary lifestyle. But it's also a fact that most people do not consume the five to seven servings a day of fruits and vegetables that are recommended to prevent cancer, heart disease, and other degenerative diseases. You simply need to adjust your carbohydrate intake to match your activity level and, within your carbohydrate strategy, choose appropriately from the carbohydrate categories.

Starting Right Now...

1. Replace high-fat foods with health-promoting carbohydrate foods. Here are some practical examples:

- Instead of adding butter or margarine to toast or bagels, use jam. Although jams contain some white sugar, most are made from whole fruits and contain added fiber (pectin and gum fiber), which can help keep cholesterol levels down.
- Instead of high-fat potato chips and dip, nacho chips, or fried treats of this kind, try these complex carbohydrate alternatives:
  - low-fat biscuits, such as melba toast, dipped in salsa
  - baked pretzels dipped in salsa or mustard
  - low-fat popcorn (less than 1.5 grams of fat per 3 cups) with no added butter or high-fat toppings.
- As a snack between meals choose fruit, raisins or other dried fruits, a low-fat bran muffin, one-half of a plain bagel with jam, or carrot sticks.

2. Don't smother carbohydrate foods with fat. Instead, use tomato sauce on pasta and low-fat yogurt on potatoes or, better still, serve a baked potato with just pepper and chopped green onions.
3. Dilute fruit juice, adding three parts water to one part juice. Fruit juices are too heavily loaded with simple sugars to be taken straight up.
4. Whenever possible, eat carbohydrate foods high in anti-cancer, disease-preventing nutrients. Incorporate at least one Category 1 or Category 2 carbohydrate food into every meal.

Fiber

Dietary fiber plays an important role in the prevention of many cancers, cardiovascular diseases, and excess weight gain. Un-fortunately, the average North American consumes only about a third of the fiber needed to help prevent these conditions.

In response to the growing public awareness of the importance of fiber, the food industry has introduced an increasing number of high-fiber breakfast cereals, crackers, and other products. This awareness can be directly attributed to the pioneering research of Doctor D. Burkitt and fellow researchers who suggested that the high-fiber diet of Africans was directly linked to their strong resistance to cancer, diabetes, heart disease, strokes, hemorrhoids, and varicose veins. This research sparked the interest of other scientists, who investigated the specific health benefits of dietary fiber. In the past 25 years, a wealth of knowledge has grown out of their efforts.

Dietary fiber is found only in the earth's vegetation. No food of animal origin contains fiber. There is no fiber in red meat, poultry, fish, dairy products, or eggs. Surprisingly, the important feature of fiber is that we cannot digest it. Fiber is really nothing more than long, branching chains of complex carbohydrates, strung together in such a way that our digestive systems are unable to break them apart. Although some fiber is metabolized by bacteria in the large intestine, much of it passes through the entire length of our intestines almost unaltered. It makes up the bulk of our fecal matter and plays an essential role in maintaining the health of the intestinal tract.

Unfortunately, in the last century we have learned to prefer our food, particularly our grains, heavily refined. We have become more accustomed to white rice, white breads, refined sugars, and refined breakfast cereals, all of which are practically devoid of dietary fiber. As a result, many of us suffer the consequences of fiber deficiency, setting ourselves up for heart disease, excess weight gain, and colon and rectal problems. Our increasingly high-fat, low-fiber diet has contributed to the fact that colon-rectal cancer is the second-leading cancer killer in North America when the statistics for men and women are combined.

Two Different Types of Dietary Fiber

Scientists have discovered many different types of fiber and have given them specific technical names, like pectin, guar gum, lignin, cellulose, and hemi-cellulose. A simpler approach is to classify these fibers according to their effects in your body: they are either cholesterol crunchers or colon cleaners. Some carbohydrate foods contain high amounts of cholesterol-cruncher fiber, which helps to lower high blood cholesterol and regulate blood sugar levels. Other carbohydrate foods contain more colon-cleaner fiber, which helps protect against cancer of the colon and rectum, and prevent irritable bowel syndrome, constipation and other bowel conditions.

Cholesterol Crunchers—As is well known, elevated cholesterol can clog your arteries over time. Clogged arteries can lead to heart attacks, strokes, and kidney failure. These cardiovascular diseases account for approximately 50 percent of all health-related deaths in our society. Keeping your cholesterol under control now can keep your from joining this statistic later.

Some complex carbohydrates contain the types of fibers that cling like magnets to cholesterol in the intestinal tract; they stop it from being absorbed into the bloodstream where it could do damage. Instead, these cholesterol crunchers drag cholesterol through the large bowel and eliminate it in the feces. They eliminate bile acids in the same way.

After a meal, bile acids are secreted by the gallbladder to aid in fat digestion. These bile acids tend to be reabsorbed into the body and converted into cholesterol by the liver. The presence of cholesterol crunchers in the intestine stops the absorption of bile acids and promotes their elimination.

An average fasting blood cholesterol level for North Americans is approximately 215-225 milligrams per hundred milli-liters of blood—or 215-225 mg percent as it is commonly expressed (in Systeme internnal units, 5.85 millimoles per liter of blood, or 5.85 mmol/liter). In a society where 50 percent of people die from cardiovascular disease, the average cholesterol level is obviously not a healthy benchmark. To be safe, you should strive for a blood cholesterol level below 200 mg percent (5.2 mmol/ liter). The safest range seems to be between 150 and 160 mg percent (3.9-4.16 mmol/liter).

If your fasting blood cholesterol level is 260 mg percent (6.76 mmol/liter), you are only nine percent above the average, but that margin will double your risk of heart attack. By simply eating one tablespoon of oat bran every day, you can reduce that 260 mg percent to 225, cutting your risk in half. Studies have proven that adding cholesterol crunchers to your daily diet can lower blood cholesterol levels, by 10 to 15 percent on average (and up to 25 percent in some cases). This can mean the difference between life and death.

Cholesterol crunchers also slow down the rate at which carbo-hydrates in the intestinal tract are absorbed into the bloodstream. Refined carbohydrates such as white sugar, brown sugar, and honey are absorbed into your bloodstream very quickly, which puts undue stress on your liver and pancreas. Cholesterol crunchers help to regulate blood sugar levels.

Finally, they make you feel full, discouraging you from overeating. Cholesterol crunchers will deliver a feeling of satiety faster than any other food except fat—which is not a good way to achieve satiety. To prove this to yourself, eat two apples or a banana or a grapefruit (about 120 calories) the next time you feel hungry between meals. By eating these satiety-producing fruits, you will almost immediately overcome the temptation to eat sweet or rich foods.

Foods High in Cholesterol Crunchers

The carbohydrate foods that contain the richest supply of cholesterol cruncher fiber are:

- oat bran, oatmeal, and oats;
- psyllium husk fiber (the main ingredient in Metamucil);
- apples, peaches, pears, and plums;
- berries (strawberries, raspberries, blackberries, boysenberries, etc.);
- white rind of citrus fruits (the white layer under the skin of oranges, grapefruits, tangerines, etc.);
- carrots;
- peas and beans, especially chickpeas and kidney beans;
- pumpernickel bread;
- ground flaxseeds, or flaxseed powder, as it is sometimes marketed (but not flaxseed oil).

"Apples, peaches, pears, and plums/Tell me when your birthday comes." Recite this childhood rhyme three times and you'll never forget which fruits are high in cholesterol crunchers.

Colon Cleaners—Colon cleaners form the second family of dietary fiber. Like cholesterol crunchers, colon cleaners are not digested or absorbed in the intestinal tract. However, they play a different role in the large intestines. Colon cleaners have been shown to help reduce the risk of colon cancer and promote better regularity of bowel function.

Acting like a sponge, colon cleaners soak up water in the intestinal tract. As a result, the fecal matter formed in the intestinal tract has a high water content, which dilutes the concentration of any toxic wastes and cancer-causing agents that may be present. Generally, the higher the concentration of cancer-causing agents, the greater the likelihood that they will cause genetic damage to the cells that line your colon and rectum.

The sponge-like colon cleaners absorb water, expanding the bulk of fecal matter. This expansion exerts a physical pressure against the inside walls of the intestinal tract, which in turn stimulates synchronized contractions of the muscular layers of the intestinal walls. These muscular contractions propel the fecal matter through the intestinal tract and out of the body, decreasing the time your intestines, colon, and rectum are exposed to cancer-causing agents. To improve the function of colon cleaners, you must drink enough water to take advantage of their sponge-like behavior. Six to eight 8-ounce glasses of water every day is widely recommended. You should also be sure to have frequent bowel movements. One per day is excellent; five per week is acceptable; having three or fewer per week is dangerous. An additional benefit is that the high water content of stools formed by colon cleaners makes them soft and easy to eliminate. They require minimal straining and are therefore less likely to cause hemorrhoids and varicose veins. (You will know your stools are sufficiently high in water content if they float.) Rock-hard, pellet-like stools are solid evidence that you lack sufficient colon-cleaner fiber to protect you from one of the most common life-threatening cancers of our day, one that is clearly related to diet.

Where do the cancer-causing agents in the intestinal tract come from? It has been known for some time that protein foods containing nitrates and nitrites, such as bacon, pepperoni, salami, hot dogs, most packaged meats, and most cold cuts, encourage the development of cancer in the colon and rectum. When the protein in these processed meats reacts with the nitrate and nitrite preservatives during digestion, carcinogenic nitrosamines are formed. These nitrosamine chemicals are only one type of cancer-causing agent against which the body must defend itself daily.

When you eat fats, your liver and gallbladder secrete bile acids into the intestine. Bile acids that are not absorbed back into the body as cholesterol remain in the intestinal tract. These can be converted into cancer-causing agents by the bacteria that line the large intestine. In this way, a diet that is high in fats contributes to the development of colon cancer by stimulating an increased secretion of bile acids. These acids can also be converted into secondary sterols (lithocholic acid and deoxycholic acid) by the bacteria in the large intestine. Secondary sterols promote rapid division of colon cells and can directly damage their genetic DNA structure. Both of these actions increase the chances of colon cancer development.

In North America one in 16 women and one in 15 men develop colon cancer. The incidence of colon cancer in parts of the world where fewer animal fats and more fiber-rich carbohydrates (especially whole grains and beans) are consumed shows as much as a 90 percent lower occurrence of this disease. Most cases of colon cancer could be prevented through healthier diet and lifestyle practices.

Other sources of carcinogens that are known to increase our risk of colon cancer:

- Alcohol generates free radicals—which can cause DNA mutations—and is a co-carcinogen, meaning it drives other cancer-causing agents into our cells with a greater efficiency. Having two or more alcoholic drinks per day is associated with a two- to three-fold increase in the risk of colon cancer, according to several prospective studies (including the Health Professionals Follow Up Study and the Nurses' Health Study).

- Heterocyclic amines are a hazard of barbecuing meat, chicken, or fish; they are formed when fat drips down onto the coals below the grill, and smoke rises from the coals. The smoke contains heterocyclic amines, known to cause cancer. They are also present in smoked meats and smoked fish, including smoked turkey, smoked salmon, and smoked chicken.

Your intestine is loaded with cancer-causing material and needs the help of colon-cleaner fiber. It is essential to consume a sufficient amount every day from the carbohydrate foods or supplements (flaxseed powder, wheat germ, and psyllium husk fiber) that are the best sources of this important protective nutrient.

Foods High in Colon Cleaners

The carbohydrate foods that supply the highest levels of colon cleaners are:

- wheat bran, including whole wheat bread and biscuits, bran cereals, wheat germ;
- rice bran, including brown rice, puffed rice and whole rice crackers;
- corn bran, corn on the cob, popcorn, cornmeal, puffed corn cereals, and corn flakes;
- peas and beans, especially chickpeas and kidney beans;
- high-fiber breakfast cereals (except oatmeal);
- psyllium husk fiber (the main ingredient in Metemucil);
- ground flaxseed or flaxseed powder (but not flaxseed oil).

Fiber in Your Diet

Keeping track of your daily fiber intake will be easy if you consult the Fiber Scoreboard on page 307. I have assigned points to each food according to its fiber content. A medium apple, for example, scores one point; one point equals three grams of dietary fiber. In order to take full advantage of colon cleaners and cholesterol crunchers, you should try to attain eight to 15 fiber points from a variety of foods every day.

Starting Right Now...

1. As you eat foods high in cholesterol crunchers, imagine that they are magnets, dragging the cholesterol and saturated fats through your intestinal tract and out of your body.

2. As you eat foods high in colon cleaners, envision them acting like a vacuum cleaner, sucking the carcinogens and other toxins from the walls of your bowels.

3. If you are indulging in a high-cholesterol food, be sure to eat a food high in cholesterol crunchers at the same time. The combination reduces the amount of cholesterol that will be absorbed into your bloodstream.

4. Drink six to eight glasses of water every day. Plenty of water is necessary for colon cleaners to work at their optimal effectiveness.

5. Make sure you are having a bowel movement at least five times a week and check that your stools float. If they do not, drink more water. Pay attention to how your bowel movements are affected by your diet. Get to know your own body rhythms.

6. If foods alone are not providing the fiber you need, take two to three teaspoons of psyllium husk fiber each day (for example, Metamucil mixed in water). Psyllium husk fiber is an excellent source of both cholesterol cruncher and colon-cleaner fiber, and has been shown to reduce high cholesterol levels in controlled clinical trials. Wheat germ also contains respectable amounts of colon-cleaner fiber.

7. Try to eat more Category 3 carbohydrates than Category 4 carbohydrates, when you are choosing grains and wheat products. For example, eat brown rice instead of white rice and whole wheat bread instead of white bread. Every gram of fiber you consume adds up to healthier bowel function in the long run.

8. Avoid processed meats, including hot dogs, bacon, pepperoni, salami, most packaged meats, and most cold cuts. They are full of saturated fats and cancer-causing preservatives.

9. I suggest that you consume two heaping tablespoons of flaxseed powder (ground organic flaxseeds) per day, about a 50-gram serving. Flaxseeds contain both cholesterol cruncher and colon-cleaner fibers, along with important natural agents that help defend against reproductive organ cancers (breast and prostate), as well as liver and gallbladder disease.

Fats

The high level of animal fat in the North American diet is the number one nutritional cause of heart attack, stroke, certain types of cancer, and obesity. This is no exaggeration. The American and Canadian heart associations, cancer associations, diabetic associations, and the National Institutes of Health in the United States have for years strongly recommended reducing our total fat intake, especially animal fats.

Many health-conscious people are concerned about white sugar in their diets. They fail to recognize that excess animal fat consumption is much more serious than eating sugar. Bacon and eggs for breakfast, pastries for dessert, large slabs of butter melting over a baked potato, cheddar cheese smothering a plate of nachos, processed meats from the local deli: these high-fat foods are the primary dietary killers in our society today. They clog your arteries, overstimulate your hormonal system, and increase the risk of cancers in the reproductive organs, the colon, and rectum.

The scientific evidence is so convincing that the department of the Surgeon General of the United States, always extremely conservative, released a Report on Nutrition and Health in July 1988 presenting its first comprehensive review of the evidence that links diet to chronic disease. The report recognized that the most common nutrition-related health problems among people in the United States were due to obesity and unbalanced diets. It identified a reduction in the consumption of fat, especially saturated fat, as the primary dietary priority for improving overall health.

Not only is eating a lot of animal fat related directly to heart disease and some cancers, but it is the major cause of obesity. Your body stores saturated fat from high-fat animal meat and dairy products very efficiently. Digesting, absorbing, transporting, and storing the fat you eat uses up only seven percent of its initial calories. In other words, your body delivers the saturated fat from your diet and stores it in your fat cells with an efficiency rate of 93 percent. When you eat saturated fat you get fat, especially if you have a slow metabolism and reduced muscle mass.

On the other hand, not all fats are bad, and it is essential to eat some fat every day to stay healthy. Certain types of fat, such as the omega-3 fats found in fish, will help protect you from heart disease, stroke, and various cancers. The predominant fat found in olive oil, canola oil, and peanut oil offers similar benefits. There are also some medicinal fats that I recommend be taken each day in a dietary supplement that contains borage seed oil, flaxseed oil, and a high-yield fish oil.

So how much fat is ideal to prevent disease and anti-aging? A few nutrition fanatics insist that you should eat nothing but grains, vegetables, tofu, and brewers' yeast, thus limiting your fat intake to 10 to15 percent of your total daily calories. This type of program is very difficult to follow and is unnecessarily restrictive for most of the population. A growing body of evidence indicates that you can take as much as 25 percent of your total calories from fat without promoting cardiovascular disease, cancer, or obesity. However, I urge you to limit your fat intake to 15 to 20 percent of your total calories each day. Populations that average fat intakes in this range tend to enjoy extraordinary health and longevity. The exceptions are the Inuit of the far north, whose diet that is 35 to 40 percent fat, most of it omega-3 fat from fish. It seems that the consumption of saturated fats from animal products and the consumption of fried foods cause most of the damage to our bodies that are attributable to fat. These sources set us up for weight gain, high cholesterol, cancer, heart disease, and gall bladder disease, whereas other fats are safer and can actually be health-promoting if consumed in the proper quantities.

The Four Families of Fat

Knowing how much fat is enough is more complicated than determining the ideal total intake. The fat in your diet is made up of four different types, or families: saturated fats, polyunsaturated fats, monounsaturated fats, and omega-3 fats (a special type of polyunsaturated fat). You need the proper amount of each family of fat because each affects your health and risk of disease in different ways. A realistic approach to achieving a healthy balance is to get approximately one-third of your fat calories from saturated fats, one-third from monounsaturated fats, and one-third from polyunsaturated and omega-3 fats. In reality, your body has no requirement at all for saturated fat, which does the most damage of all the fats. But the only way to avoid all saturated fat is to become a vegan vegetarian, eating no animal products at all, and strictly avoiding chocolate, palm oil, and coconut oil. Vegans tend have a reduced risk of many degenerative diseases, but few individuals are willing to go to this extreme. Most want to consume some meat and dairy foods as part of their lifestyle, and for them I have developed a program that allows these foods, while keeping the amount of saturated fats within a safe range.

Saturated Fats—Let's look first at this most dangerous family of dietary fat—saturated fats. I've recommended that roughly one third of your total fat intake be saturated fats. Adapting this discipline is one of the most important steps you can take in preventing obesity and cardiovascular and other degenerative diseases.

Foods High in Saturated Fats

- sour cream, butter, whole milk, cream, ice cream, 2% milk and yogurt;

- cheese that is more than three percent milk fat—that's almost every cheese, including cheddar, blue, brick, colby, cream, muenster and port du salut;

- egg yolks;

- all red meats, all pork products, many processed luncheon meats (hot dogs, salami, bologna, prosciutto, corned beef, pastrami, spare ribs, bacon), and organ meats (liver, kidney, brains);

- chocolate (cocoa butter), coconut oil, palm oil;

- baked goods and candy made with palm oil or palm kernel oil.

Saturated fats interact with cholesterol to give you double trouble. Surprisingly, it's not necessarily the cholesterol in food that elevates your blood cholesterol levels. Up to two-thirds of the cholesterol in your body is produced by your liver; only one-third comes from the cholesterol you eat, unless you are eating a lot of egg yolks and organ meats. Elevated blood cholesterol is most often a result of eating too much saturated fat. When you ingest saturated fat, it is absorbed from your intestines, then carried to your liver, where it stimulates cholesterol production. The more saturated fat you eat, the more cholesterol your liver produces.

Coconut oil and palm oil, used in commercially made baked goods, don't contain any cholesterol at all, but they are heavily loaded with saturated fat. It's their saturated fat content that makes them ideal for baking: they are very stable when heated to high temperatures. When these saturated fats enter your body as ingredients in cookies, pie crust, and other pastries, they are transported to your liver, where they switch on that organ's cholesterol manufacturing machine. Chocolate can have the same effect. Chocolate contains no cholesterol but is high in saturated fat content. Beware of foods advertised as being cholesterol-free: this doesn't mean they won't increase the level of cholesterol in your blood.

The situation is worse if you eat foods that contain high levels of both saturated fat and cholesterol. These are found together only in foods of animal origin; cholesterol is produced solely in the tissues of animals (including fish and seafood), not plants.

A Double Whammy: Foods High in Saturated Fat and Cholesterol

- whole milk products (chocolate milk, whole milk yogurt, heavy cream);
- high-fat cheeses, ice cream, butter;
- mayonnaise, egg yolks (not egg whites);
- organ meats (liver, brains, sweetbreads, kidney, heart);
- red meats and pork (for example, hamburgers, steak, pork, lamb and veal, sausage);
- bacon, most cold cuts with the exception of chicken and turkey breast.

Cholesterol, Heart Disease and Cancer

How does cholesterol contribute to the threat of heart disease, strokes, and certain types of cancer? The process is really quite remarkable. One of your liver's primary functions is to transport saturated fat to other tissues of the body. This task is not an easy one because fats can't dissolve in your bloodstream; it's a physiological demonstration of the old saying, "Oil and water don't mix." The liver therefore repackages the fat with other, more soluble substances before sending it through your bloodstream: it builds, in effect, a miniature "shuttle bus." The outer frame of the shuttle bus is made up of protein. The inside is filled with saturated fat and cholesterol.

Once the bus is full, it is sealed and sent out of the liver to enter the bloodstream. The outer protein shell of the bus allows part of the fat and cholesterol to dissolve and float freely. As the shuttle bus passes by muscles, it opens its doors and allows some fat to be taken up. As a rule, when your muscles are not working vigorously, they prefer to burn fat, thus preserving their stores of carbohydrates for use as high-octane fuel during strenuous exercise. (Your heart muscle in particular likes to burn fat for energy.) The shuttle bus eventually delivers any remaining saturated fat to your fat cells. Too many deliveries, and the fat cells become enlarged; you begin to look overweight.

But what about the cholesterol in the shuttle bus? It too is delivered to your cells. In the adrenal glands, cholesterol is used to make hormones like cortisone. In the ovaries, it is used to make estrogen and progesterone. In the male testes, it is the building block of the male hormone testosterone. Cholesterol is also necessary for the creation of bile acids, vitamin D, and the fatty, waxy membrane around the outside of every body cell. Your body needs a certain amount of cholesterol to remain healthy. However, when you consume a diet high in saturated fat and/or cholesterol, the shuttle buses transport more cholesterol than your cells require for normal functioning. The shuttle bus doors will open and allow excess cholesterol to exit into the bloodstream, where it will stick to the inside lining of the blood vessel walls. This causes the arteries to narrow, and eventually restricts the circulation of blood.

This narrowing process, known as atherosclerosis—hardening or narrowing of the arteries—is the major contributing cause of heart disease, stroke, and related cardiovascular diseases. When less blood and oxygen circulates to the heart muscle, the result is an angina episode or a heart attack. A lack of oxygen in the brain cells can bring on an ischemic stroke or cause the vessels to become rigid, losing their elasticity. Then they are more easily ruptured, resulting in a hemorrhagic stroke.

The cholesterol that is left in your arteries by the LDL-cholesterol shuttle bus forms the main component of thickening arterial plaque. Once an artery becomes almost completely obstructed by plaque, you are a prime candidate for a heart attack, stroke, or even kidney failure. Unfortunately, arterial narrowing due to plaque is invisible and painless until the final stages. Death by heart attack or stroke can happen suddenly, with no warning signs.

Almost fifty percent of North Americans die of cardiovascular diseases, most of them as a result of obstructed and rigid arteries. Just because you can't see it or feel it doesn't mean you should ignore it. If you are lucky, you will experience an early alarm—the squeezing chest and arm pain of angina. For at least 25 percent of those people with advanced blood vessel narrowing, though, a fatal heart attack is their first and last symptom of heart disease.

To make matters worse, some evidence suggests that excess cholesterol delivered to your fat tissues, adrenal glands, ovaries, and testes may overstimulate the production of certain hormones, such as estrogen and testosterone. Imbalances in these reproductive hormones have been associated with an increased risk of breast cancer, prostate cancer, and other cancers of the reproductive organs.

When I caution people about the health risks associated with eating high-fat red meats, pork products, cheese, and other foods loaded with saturated fat, they often respond by saying that it's not a problem for them. They burn off the fat with exercise, which prevents them from gaining weight.

True, you can burn off the fat calories with exercise; however, you cannot burn off the cholesterol your body produces to transport saturated fats through your bloodstream. Every mouthful of saturated fat stimulates cholesterol production in your liver, and if you manufacture more cholesterol than your body needs, it is most likely lodging inside your artery walls. Even marathon-level training and fitness cannot adequately protect your arteries if you consume too much saturated fat.

How much is too much? According to experts like Dr. William Castelli, M.D., for many years the scientific director of the Framingham Heart Study, more than 15 to 20 grams of saturated fat per day puts you at risk for elevated cholesterol, no matter what exercise program you follow. Note that the average intake of saturated fat in North America per day is 70 to 80 grams. The program that I will outline will keep your average saturated fat intake at five to 15 grams per day.

There is no way to win with saturated fat. Even if you have great genetics and your body is able to efficiently clear excess cholesterol from your bloodstream, you are still putting yourself at risk for colon cancer and possibly reproductive organ cancers as well.

Now for a bit of good news: not all cholesterol contributes to a hardening of your arteries. Up to this point, we have been watching only the LDL cholesterol shuttle bus. The liver makes a high-density lipoprotein (HDL) cholesterol shuttle bus, which it also releases to the bloodstream. This vehicle actually vacuums up deposits of LDL cholesterol from your artery walls and carries that cholesterol back to your liver. There it can be used for other purposes, such as producing bile acids. (Of course, if you are still eating foods high in saturated fats and cholesterol, your liver will have too much cholesterol already and will just send it back out to your arteries again.)

Studies have shown that people with high levels of HDL cholesterol (the good guys) and low levels of LDL cholesterol (the bad guys) are much less likely to experience heart attacks or the advanced stages of atherosclerosis. Some recent research has confirmed that raising levels of HDL cholesterol can actually reverse hardening of arteries that has already occurred. Certainly, the ratio of LDL to HDL cholesterol levels can tell your doctor a lot about your chances of developing cardiovascular disease. Next time you are having blood work done, ask to see where you stand. But even if your LDL-to-HDL ratio is low, remember that it is easier to cut back on saturated fat and cholesterol now rather than wait until the damage is done.

Allowable Sources of Saturated Fat

- Chicken, turkey, and Cornish hens
- Cheese that is under 4% milk fat
- Skim milk and 1% milk
- Non-fat and 1% yogurt

Polyunsaturated Fats—Unlike saturated fats, polyunsaturated fats are essential for good health. Early studies showed that corn oil, a substance high in polyunsaturated fats, could lower blood cholesterol levels. However, we know today that some polyunsaturated oils may present more dangers to your health than benefits. First, polyunsaturated fats contain many unstable bonds between constituent atoms that allow them to be easily converted into cancer-causing free radicals when heated to high temperatures (by deep frying or pan frying, for example).

Animal studies have shown that a diet rich in certain polyunsaturated fats (corn oil and other vegetable oils high in linoleic acid) increases the incidence of cancerous tumors when these unsaturated fats are combined with carcinogens, then fed to animals with transplanted tumors or to animals that have been bred to express a genetic vulnerability to a certain type of cancer. By contrast, lower tumor incidences in the same studies were associated with consumption of omega-3 fats (from fish or flaxseed oil), and in some cases the consumption of monounsaturated fats (often from olive oil). It seems that certain unsaturated fats may increase our risk of cancer, through their conversion to a hormone known as prostaglandin hormone series-2. This prostaglandin hormone increases the replication rate of cells in the body, which increases the chances of genetic mutations occurring.

A second threat develops from the tendency of certain polyunsaturated fats to become the building block of a chemical called thromboxane. Thromboxane prompts the blood platelets to stick together more readily than normal, resulting in clogged arteries and inflammation in the artery walls. In addition, thromboxane encourages the arteries to go into spasm, contributing to further narrowing.

If you want to keep your blood vessels open and minimize your risk of heart disease or stroke, keep the amount of thromboxane you produce from polyunsaturated fats as low as possible. I recommend that you avoid corn oil, sunflower seed oil, safflower oil, and soybean oil, along with mixed vegetable oils and the products made from them.

Avoid Foods High in Polyunsaturated Fat

- most vegetable oils, including corn oil, sunflower seed oil, soybean oil, and safflower oil;
- partially hydrogenated foods, such as margarine, shortening, and processed peanut butter.

Partially hydrogenated foods, such as margarine, vegetable shortening, and processed peanut butter, can be especially dangerous. These foods are made from polyunsaturated fats that have been made more concentrated. Although this process gives them a solid consistency and greater "spreadability," the body has difficulty absorbing partially hydrogenated polyunsaturated fats; it does not know what they are. Recent studies have demonstrated that hydrogenated fats raise cholesterol levels just as saturated fats do. These fats also encourage the formation of thromboxane and other potentially harmful substances. They are best avoided or kept to a minimum.

Monounsaturated Fats—The third family of fats is composed of monounsaturated fats, found mainly in olive oil, peanut oil, and canola oil. These fats help lower cholesterol but are much more stable than polyunsaturated fats when exposed to heat, air, and light. They are not easily converted into free radicals. Mediterranean and Asian civilizations have relied on olive oil and peanut oil as their main sources of dietary fat for thousands of years. In general, people from these cultures have less risk of heart disease and certain forms of cancer than North Americans. We know less about rapeseed oil, commonly known as canola oil, because it is a relative newcomer to our tables. However, recent research suggests that it provides the same benefits as olive oil and peanut oil. Conveniently, all three contain small amounts of polyunsaturated fats. Your body does need some polyunsaturated fats, but not the excess found in corn oil and related polyunsaturated fat oils.

Some new evidence suggests that olive oil can help to lower blood pressure and improve the regulation of blood sugars, as well as to reduce levels of cholesterol in the blood. Considering all these features, olive oil, peanut oil, and canola oil should become the main sources of oil in your diet. Approximately one-third of your total dietary fat intake can consist of monounsaturated fats. Use them for salad dressings, to sauté vegetables, to make stir-fry dishes, or to brown poultry.

The Benefits of Olive Oil and Peanut Oil

- they help lower the level of cholesterol in your blood;
- they help lower your blood pressure;
- they improve the regulation of blood sugar;
- they are not as carcinogenic when exposed to light, heat, or oxygen as polyunsaturated vegetable oils are, and they do not make your blood sticky;
- they help maintain levels of HDL (the good cholesterol).

About Nuts, Seeds and Avocados—Many nuts, seeds, and avocados contain monounsaturated fat, but they deliver large amounts of all types of fat, which can easily contribute to weight gain and obesity. When it comes to monounsaturated fats, your body benefits from small quantities, such as a teaspoon of olive oil in salad dressing. Although it is a healthier fat, it is still fat, and any excess fat calories you consume will be delivered to your fat cells to be stored. You can eat avocados occasionally, but don't make them a frequent addition to your meals. It is best to avoid nuts, seeds, and olives, unless you are a vegan vegetarian consuming no meat or dairy products at all. A small snack of mixed nuts and seeds is a better option than chocolate bars or doughnuts, but don't make them a regular part of your diet. You just don't need that much total fat.

Omega-3 Fats—The fourth family of fats are the omega-3 fats, a special type of polyunsaturated fat found in fish and seafood. In general, the higher the fat content of the fish, the greater the amount of omega-3 fats. Flaxseed oil also contains a unique omega-3 fat called alpha-linolenic acid, which provides health benefits similar to those of the omega-3 fats from fish and seafood.

Fish and Seafood Especially High in Omega-3 Fats

- anchovies, clams, crab, halibut, herring, mackerel, mullet, mussels, red snapper, rockfish, salmon, sardines, shad, swordfish, trout, tuna

Some populations, such as the Inuit and those in Japan who live in fishing villages, enjoy especially low incidences of heart disease and cancer. Research findings suggest that people who rely substantially on fish, particularly fatty fish, as their main source of protein have significantly reduced risks of heart disease, related cardiovascular conditions, colon cancer, and cancers of the reproductive organs, compared to populations that consume lower quantities of omega-3 fats. Inuit who have migrated to southern Canada and Japanese who have moved to North America soon find that if they adopt the typical North American diet, high in saturated fats, their incidence of cardiovascular disease and cancer becomes the same as ours.

Omega-3 fats seem to lower blood cholesterol levels significantly when they are substituted for foods high in saturated fats. Preliminary intervention studies have shown that when individuals with high levels of cholesterol in their blood eat more fatty fish, their cholesterol levels are reduced. Omega-3 fats also make the blood less likely to form abnormal clots on the inside of blood vessel walls, thanks largely to their conversion into prostaglandin series-3 hormones within the cells of the cardiovascular system. Omega-3 fats are the building blocks of prostaglandin series-3 hormones, which reduce the stickiness of blood platelets and abnormal clotting of the blood. That clotting is a frequently encountered lethal step towards a heart attack or ischemic stroke.

Because of these benefits of omega-3 fats, I encourage the frequent consumption of fish and the occasional consumption of seafood. Note that seafood—clams, mussels, shrimp, lobster, and crab—contains higher amounts of cholesterol than most fish. However, if your cholesterol is normal (below 200 mg percent; 5.2 mmol/liter) and you do not have established heart disease, then substituting seafood once or twice a month is perfectly acceptable in my view.

Fighting the Fat Temptation—Without a doubt, foods that are high in fat, especially saturated fat, are considered the most delicious and satisfying in our diets. From my experience with patients, the greatest dietary challenge tends to be cutting back on the amount of unhealthy fat they eat. It is also the most important and life-enhancing change you can make in your eating habits. It's up to you to start overcoming the fat temptations in your life.

I know you're going to indulge in butter, pastries, mayonnaise, or ice cream from time to time. It's almost impossible not to—and it's not the end of the world. It's what you regularly do on most days that really matters. Keep making wellness choices from moment to moment. With time, you will have fewer and fewer setbacks.

Make a commitment to yourself now to cut back on the amount of bad fat you eat. Then make these promises a reality. Know that saturated fat from animal products and fried foods is your number one health enemy.

Natural Supplements That Lower Cholesterol and Triglycerides

If your cholesterol is already high (above 200 mg percent or 5.2 mmol/liter), it is extremely important to keep your saturated fat and cholesterol intake down by consistently choosing the carbohydrate foods that provide cholesterol-cruncher fiber. In addition, there are two outstanding natural supplements that are proven to reduce high cholesterol levels without producing adverse side effects. These natural cholesterol-lowering agents are gum guggul and policosanol.

As you know, the statin drugs that are often prescribed to lower cholesterol are known to cause liver damage, and thus require the monitoring of liver enzymes in those who use them. Other side effects of these drugs include fatigue, upset stomach, gas, constipation, and abdominal pain and cramps. In rare cases muscle pain can occur, and may progress to a life-threatening condition known as rhabdomyolysis. Statin drugs, which block the synthesis of cholesterol in the liver, include lovastatin (prescription name: Mevacor), pravastatin (Pravachol), simvastin (Zocor), fluvastatin sodium (Lescol, Lescol XL), atorvastatin calcium (Lipitor), and rosuvastatin (Crestor).

Such drugs are often unnecessary. The same cholesterol-lowering effect can be achieved by a natural supplement that contains gum guggul and policosanol. Gum guggul (botancial name: Gugulipid) is a gummy resin derived from the mukul myrrh tree. In human clinical trials it lowered both cholesterol (which was lowered by 14 to 27 percent) and triglycerides (lowered by 22 to 33 percent) within a four- to12-week period. Gum guggul is widely prescribed in India. It has a proven safety record and is very non-toxic. Occasional side effects include minor intestinal upset, skin rash, diarrhea, and nausea.

Policosanol is a natural substance found in sugar cane; it can also be produced from beeswax. It has been shown to lower LDL-cholesterol up to 24 percent and to increase HDL—results that were superior to the statin drugs it was tested against in human subjects with high cholesterol problems. Like gum guggul, policosanol does not damage the liver and produces only mild side effects on rare occasions. At high doses (above 10 mg per day) it can act as an anti-coagulant, so daily doses above 10 mg should not be combined with other anti-coagulant drugs—Aspirin, warfarin, Coumadin, Plavix—unless monitoring of bleeding time (or prothrombin time) is routinely performed by a physician.

I have formulated a cholesterol-lowering supplement which I make available to my patients and other health professionals. It contains, in one capsule, 500 mg (standardized to 2.5 percent guggulsterone content) gum guggul and 1.75 mg policosanol. Individuals with high cholesterol are directed to take three to six capsules per day (one or two capsules, three times per day). These two natural agents have been largely overlooked by Western medicine, but their effectiveness and safety profile make them an excellent intervention to help lower cholesterol in individuals whose diet and exercise are not enough to keep cholesterol and triglyceride levels within a safe range.

Starting Right Now...

1. When you consume high-fat animal foods—red meat, pork, organ meats, cheeses, pizza with cheese, cream in your coffee, sour cream or butter on your baked potato, or butter on your toast—visualize the arterial plaque that is building up on the insides of your artery walls. This visualization process is the first step in overcoming the temptation to eat high-fat, disease-promoting foods.

2. Stop using butter; it's almost pure saturated fat. Instead spread a little jam on toast and moisten sandwiches with lettuce, tomato, cucumber, or a touch of olive oil.

3. Try to avoid all foods that are high in cholesterol and saturated fat. Switch to low-fat dairy products (skim milk, low-fat cheeses, "light" sour cream, and low-fat yogurt) and low-fat flesh products (poultry and fish).

4. Think twice before eating foods advertised as "cholesterol-free." They may be high in saturated fat, which switches on your body's production of cholesterol. In particular, avoid products that list palm, palm kernel, or coconut oil on the list of ingredients. Remember that chocolate is also loaded with saturated fat.

5. Use margarine and processed peanut butter only occasionally, if at all. They contain partially hydrogenated fats that can elevate cholesterol levels and increase the stickiness of your blood. Even fresh made, unadulterated peanut butter is high in total fat and I do not recommend it for regular use, as is the case for eating most nuts, olives and seeds.

6. Use olive oil, canola oil, or peanut oil instead of other vegetable oils to sauté vegetables, brown chicken or turkey, in a stir-fry, and in salad dressings. Avoid corn oil, sunflower seed oil, soybean oil, safflower oil, or mixed vegetable oils.

7. Avoid any kind of deep-fried or pan-fried foods.

8. Choose varieties of fish that are especially high in omega-3 fats on regular basis.

Protein

In the Northern American diet, the major sources of dietary protein are foods of animal origin—meat, poultry, egg whites, fish, and dairy products. The secret to using protein foods in a health-promoting way is to choose those that are high in protein, but low in saturated fat and cholesterol.

The principal role of dietary protein is to provide the major framework material for your muscles, bones, teeth, hair, and nails. Protein helps build and rebuild your body's supporting tissues from day to day. It also performs other roles, such as enzyme formation, transportation of nutrients through the bloodstream, immune system functions, hormone formation, and more. Clearly, consuming the right amount of protein each day is critical to your health. In my program, 20 to 40 percent of your total calories each day are derived from protein. (Like fats and carbohydrates, protein is measured in calories even though it is not primarily used by your body as fuel.)

It's important not to overconsume protein. Overconsumption forces the body to convert some of the excess protein to saturated fat. A high protein intake also generates by-products like urea and uric acid, which can stress the kidneys and may lead to attacks of gouty arthritis in some people.

For simplicity, I have divided the allowable low-fat protein foods into two categories: low-fat flesh protein foods and low-fat dairy protein foods. Both protein sources provide high-quality protein, and each contributes other nutrients to your overall wellness store.

Protein from Low-Fat Dairy Foods

Once a day, you should have a generous serving of a low-fat dairy product such as low-fat milk, yogurt, or cheese. Almost all dairy products display the percentage of milk fat—abbreviated as "% M.F."— on the container. A low-fat cheese will be labeled 3% M.F. or less; a low-fat milk, buttermilk, or yogurt will say 1% M.F. or less. Although egg whites are not officially dairy products, I have them on the list of choices. Egg yolks contain saturated fat and 250 mg of cholesterol per egg. On any given day you should consume no more than 150 to 200 mg of cholesterol, so egg yolks are off the list. However, egg whites are an outstanding source of high-quality protein.

If you restrict your dairy intake to these products, you will help ensure that your total calories from fat will be less than 20 percent. These foods are important not only because they are high in protein and low in cholesterol, but because they contain essential minerals and vitamins, most notably calcium and vitamin D.

Low-Fat Dairy Protein Foods

- skim or 1% milk
- yogurt (1% M.F. or less)
- egg whites
- cheese with 3% M.F. or less
- buttermilk (skim or 1% M.F.)

Calcium from Low-Fat Dairy Foods

Calcium is essential to your health regardless of age. Critical to the maintenance of strong bones and teeth, it is also important for normal heart rhythm, muscle contraction, blood clotting, and the regulation of blood pressure. Preliminary evidence suggests that optimal calcium intake can help reduce high blood pressure and prevent its onset. Calcium and vitamin D may be significant in the prevention of colon cancer.

Equally vital, calcium prevents osteoporosis, a condition in which calcium is reabsorbed from the bones back into the bloodstream and then passed out of the body in urine, leaving the bones prone to fracture. In the United States alone osteoporosis affects 15 to 20 million people and accounts for 1.3 million fractures each year. It is especially prevalent among post-menopausal women. Yet osteoporosis is almost completely preventable if your calcium intake is adequate throughout your lifetime, and if you have sufficient vitamin D in your diet, remain physically active, and maintain a healthy weight. Smoking and alcohol consumption encourage osteoporosis, as do other lifestyle influences that affect bone mass.

Your daily requirement of calcium changes with age. Between 11 and 24 years of age all individuals should ingest 1200 to 1500 mg per day of calcium, a level that has been shown to optimize bone density and forestall the development of osteoporosis later in life. From ages 24 to 50, a daily intake of 1000 mg is adequate to maintain bone density in men and women. After age 50, women require about 1500 mg per day to help prevent bone loss that results from the drop-off in estrogen levels. At age 65, men should also increase their intake to 1500 mg per day, since one in eight men will develop osteoporosis after the age of 50.

The richest and most easily absorbed sources of calcium are dairy products. Numerous studies indicate that the calcium from dairy products is easily absorbed. The vitamin D in milk and most yogurt products improves the absorption of calcium from the intestines to the bloodstream still further. Insufficient blood levels of vitamin D are strongly linked to the development of osteoporosis, along with inadequate calcium intake.

One eight-ounce serving of low-fat yogurt provides 350 to 400 mg of calcium. An eight-ounce glass of milk contains about 300 mg. As for cheeses, three or four ounces of most varieties will supply 300 to 400 mg of calcium. (There are exceptions: eight ounces of cottage cheese has only 130 mg of calcium.)

Calcium is also available from complex carbohydrate sources such as green leafy vegetables (spinach, collard greens, Swiss chard), beans, peas, kale, broccoli, bread, and grain products. As a rule, most teenagers and adults fall short of their daily calcium requirement by at least 500 mg. This is why I recommend taking a high-potency multi-vitamin and mineral every day that contains 500 mg of elemental calcium and 400 IU of vitamin D. Very often additional calcium and/or vitamin D is necessary, as we'll see in the next chapter.

Calcium Levels in Common Foods

Product	Amount	Calcium (mg)
Low-fat yogurt	1 cup	415 mg
Low-fat milk	1 cup	300 mg
Low-fat cottage cheese	½ cup	75 mg
Sardines with bones	3 oz	370 mg
Salmon with bones (canned)	3 oz	165 mg
Processed tofu with calcium sulfate	4 oz	145 mg
Canned shrimp	3 oz	100 mg
Cooked lentils	1 cup	75 mg
Chicken	3 oz	10 mg
Tuna	3 oz	5 mg
Collard greens	½ cup	180 mg
Spinach	½ cup	85 mg
Stalk of broccoli	½ cup	70 mg
Orange	1 medium	55 mg
Green beans	½ cup	30 mg
Lettuce	¼ head	15 mg
Orange juice	½ cup	10 mg
Apple	1 medium	10 mg
Whole wheat bread	1 slice	20 mg
Cooked spaghetti	1 cup	15 mg
Cooked rice	½ cup	10 mg

Protein from Low-Fat Flesh Foods

Low-fat flesh provides the second source of protein with which you should be familiar. The foods in this category are not only important sources of high-quality protein and low in fat and cholesterol, they are also the major dietary sources of two very important nutrients: vitamin B12 and iron. Here is a list of low-fat protein foods:

Low-Fat Flesh Protein Foods

- chicken breast
- turkey breast
- Cornish hens
- fish
- seafood
- tofu and other soy products (e.g., soy cheese)

Vitamin B12—Vitamin B12 is an essential ingredient for the normal reproduction and replication of all your body's cells. Your cells need it to pass on precise genetic material from one generation of cells to the next. Vitamin B12 deficiency is very serious: the red blood cells become abnormally large, a condition known as megablastosis, and fail to deliver oxygen to the tissues properly. The result can be full-blown pernicious anemia. Cells with short life spans are the first to be affected by vitamin B12 deficiency. The cells that line the respiratory and intestinal tracts may need replacement after only seven to 14 days. Red blood cells live only 120 days. Severe vitamin B12 deficiency also affects the nervous system and the brain.

Flesh foods are one of the few sources of vitamin B12. Vegetarians are susceptible to vitamin B12 deficiency, because few vegetables, grains, cereals, fruits, legumes, or dairy products contain appreciable amounts.

Iron—We think of spinach and lentils as being high in iron, and indeed they are. But the presence of fiber makes the iron in plant foods difficult to absorb from the intestine into the bloodstream. The fiber will drag up to 95 percent of the iron through the intestines, where it is ultimately expelled as part of the feces. A large percentage of the iron in vegetables, cereals, and legumes is not really available to your body at all. The most easily digested sources of iron are flesh foods. This iron, called heme iron, is bound to protein, so it is easily absorbed into the bloodstream. Chicken, turkey, Cornish hen, and most fish are rich sources of dietary iron.

As a component of hemoglobin in red blood cells, iron has the vital role of transporting oxygen—picking it up from the lungs and carrying it to every cell in your body. Iron is critical for energy production and immune system functioning. Iron deficiency is the leading mineral deficiency worldwide. Up to 50 percent of all women may have at least grade one iron deficiency, because they don't get enough iron in their diets and they routinely lose it through menstruation. Grade one deficiency leads to fatigue, weakness, and a depressed immune system. In more severe cases, iron deficiency anemia may occur.

Eating two low-fat flesh foods every day, combined with a variety of vegetables, cereals, beans, and peas, will help ensure your daily iron requirement. As with calcium, additional iron (about 6 mg per day) from a high potency multi-vitamin and mineral supplement is a prudent strategy. A unique feature of iron is that the body will absorb only as much as it requires, provided you are not bombarding your system with extremely high supplemental doses. If you find yourself regularly feeling tired for no good reason, then ask your physician to check your serum ferritin levels, a sensitive indicator of early-stage iron deficiency. If iron deficiency is present, then iron supplementation with prescription-level doses (such as 300 mg, three times per day of ferrous sulfate or gluconate) is warranted.

Free Range Chicken

Although skinless chicken breast is known to be low in saturated fat and cholesterol, the commercially raised chickens we consume today are raised quite differently than chickens raised under more natural conditions. Commercially raised chickens are crammed into closed coops to conserve space and maximize profitability and fed antibiotics and hormones to increase growth and fight disease. It is difficult to assess the extent that these toxins, hormones and other drugs may have on the health of humans if they are ingested on a regular basis. Luckily, eating only skinless chicken breast reduces not only your fat intake, compared to eating other higher fat meat products, but also helps to minimize the ingestion of toxins and hormones that concentrate in the fattier part of the chicken (legs, wings, organs). Free-range chicken represents the healthiest approach to skinless chicken breast consumption. These birds are allowed to run free, which lowers their body fat concentrations, and are fed organic feed, free of pesticides, hormones and antibiotics. Their meat also contains significantly higher amounts of omega-3 fats. Free-range chicken is more expensive and is more difficult to find, but for those with bigger budgets and accessibility to these birds, it is the best way to go.

Some Precautions Regarding Fish and Seafood

Fish is generally regarded as a good source of protein, low in saturated fat and high in omega-3 fats, making it a desirable, health-promoting food. However, fish from coastal waters, particularly near large cities, have alarmingly high levels of toxin concentrations of industrial waste, sewage, pesticides, insecticides,

PCB's (polychlorinated biphenyls), DDT (dichlorodiphenyl-trichloroethane) dioxin, methyl mercury and lead. Fish tend to accumulate toxins in their fatty tissue and pass those toxins along to us when we eat them. It is best to consume cold-water species like cod, haddock, perch, salmon, dolphin-safe tuna and herring, as they thrive in the open sea, away from the polluted coastal waters. Also limit your intake of fish that consume near the top of the food chain, ingesting the toxins from smaller fish. Such fish include bluefish, carp, catfish, striped bass and trout. Even fish raised in commercial fishponds are not necessarily immune to toxins, as pesticides and herbicides from nearby fields can pollute these ponds.

With shellfish, some health authorities suggest that they are storage tanks of toxins. Shellfish found in coastal waters are reported to feed on debris and are unable to efficiently excrete toxins and pollutants through their outer hard shell casings. They concentrate these toxins and pass them up the food chain to humans upon their consumption. On the positive side, shellfish are high in protein, low in saturated fat, contain low to moderate amounts of omega-3 fats, and varying amounts of cholesterol. How much of a threat the toxins found in shellfish pose to human health is still not clear but as a precaution consume shellfish no more than once or twice a month.

Protein in Complex Carbohydrates

On my program, your principal protein intake includes one serving of a low-fat dairy food and two servings of low-fat flesh protein selections, every day. However, some carbohydrate foods also contain a supplemental amount of protein, which can help meet your daily protein requirement. In fact, most carbohydrates except fruit contain small but important amounts of protein. Especially good sources are peas, chickpeas, and beans. Potatoes, corn, rice, pasta, and many breads and cereals also provide respectable amounts of additional protein.

How Much Protein Do You Need Each Day?

The more you weigh (especially in terms of muscle mass) and the more active you are, the more protein your body requires to support its lean mass and perform other protein-dependent functions. You can calculate your protein needs by multiplying your weight in pounds by 0.4, 0.5, 0.6, 0.7, or 0.8, depending on your level of activity. To estimate your protein need in grams per day, follow these steps:

1. Review the descriptions and values of these five activity levels and determine which type most accurately reflects your current activity level.

    Sedentary: No exercise, no heavy manual work.

    Value: 0.4

    Mildly Active: Thirty minutes of fat-burning aerobic exercise five to seven times per week. No heavy manual work or resistance training.

    Value: 0.5

    Moderately Active: Thirty minutes of fat-burning aerobic exercise five to seven times per week; weight training program three or more times per week, or heavy manual labour.

    Value: 0.6

    More Advanced Activity: Minimum of 30 minutes of fat-burning aerobic exercise five to seven times per week; one hour of high-intensity weight training five or more times per week.

    Value: 0.7

    Heavy Training: More than 90 minutes of weight training five or more times per week with additional aerobic activity.

    Value: 0.8

2. Determine your activity level type from Step 1, and write its assigned value here: _____

3. Estimate your protein need in grams per day by multiplying your weight in pounds by the assigned value of your activity level type:

___ lbs. x ____ assigned value = _____

My protein requirement per day is _____

Now that you have identified your approximate protein needs in grams per day, become familiar with the number of grams of protein available from the low-fat protein foods highlighted in this section, as outlined in the table below.

It can sometimes be difficult to reach your protein goal once you factor in the increased requirements imposed by exercise. A protein shake that is low in carbohydrates (under seven grams per serving) and fat (under two grams per serving) may be the answer. I use a protein shake mix every morning that provides 25 grams of protein per scoop, less than six grams of carbohydrates and less than one gram of fat. I mix two scoops in a blender with ice cubes and two tablespoons of flaxseed powder. This provides me with 50 grams of protein to start my day, which makes it much easier to achieve the required total daily intake of 130 to 140 grams.

You have to be more careful with protein bars, as they contain higher quantities of refined sugars in addition to the grams of protein they provide. Protein bars can promote weight gain because the sugars will be converted to fat if your body does not need the carbohydrate calories at the time of consumption. Protein bars should be used more as a meal replacement when you've had to skip a meal and find yourself feeling hypoglycemic.

Protein Foods with Little Fat

Food Portion	Grams of Protein
Chicken 3 oz.	27
Turkey 3 oz.	28
Chicken ¼ broiled	22.4
Most fish 3 oz.	20
Tuna ½ cup	15.9
Tuna 3 oz.	24
Kidney beans ½ cup	7.5
Corn ½ cup	2.5
Green peas ½ cup	4.0
White bread 1 slice	2.0
Typical breakfast cereal 1 serving	2 – 4
Tomatoes 1 medium	1.0
Most fruits 1 serving	0.3 – 0.8
Pasta 1 cup cooked	7
Oysters 6 medium	15.1
Egg white - 1	7
Dairy cottage cheese 5-6 tbsp.	19.5
1% yogurt or 1% milk 8 oz.	8.5
Soy milk low-fat 8 oz.	4
Soy cheese low-fat 1 oz.	7
Rice ½ cup cooked	2.0
Green beans ½ cup	1.0
Baked potato 1 medium	3.0
Whole wheat bread 1 slice	3.0
Saltines 4 crackers	1.0
Banana 1 medium	1.1
Bagel 1 medium	7

Starting Right Now...

1. Eat only one serving of a low-fat dairy food and two servings of a low-fat flesh food every day. The size of the servings will depend on your body size and activity level, and thus your total daily protein need.

2. Collect recipes for preparing low-fat flesh and dairy foods such as chicken, fish, and low-fat cheese. Often you can adapt your favorite recipes by cutting back on the fat and making simple substitutions.

Water and Other Fluids

This is the fifth nutritional component in your diet: water and fluids. Many of us walk around every day in a semi-dehydrated state, yet nearly every chemical reaction that takes place in our bodies requires water. This is why dehydration can lead to death so quickly. All of the essential life processes shut down when you are severely dehydrated.

To ensure that your body functions at its best, drink six to eight glasses (1.5 to 2 quarts or litres) of water or other fluids every day. Of course, intensive, prolonged exercise demands an even greater intake of fluids. Maintaining enough water in your bloodstream is necessary for transporting nutrients to your tissues and for pushing your blood through the kidneys. Even partial dehydration will impair your kidneys' ability to filter toxins and waste products from your blood.

Water is important for improving your metabolic efficiency and for burning fat in your tissue cells. If you don't drink enough water, you can hinder the fat-burning process. Water also flushes excess sodium out of your body. Higher sodium levels are linked to high blood pressure in some people. Diuretic foods—foods that increase urine output—will likewise help your body eliminate unwanted sodium. All fruits and vegetables in their natural states (not canned or processed) are diuretic foods, but these foods are effective only if you drink enough water each day.

Too Much Salt—Food manufacturers add sodium to everything we eat, from pickles to pancake mix. Most North Americans consume between 1600 and 2300 mg of sodium per day from commercially processed foods alone. They pick up another 1200 mg from the sodium that occurs naturally in food. Then they consume a further 1300 to 2500 mg when they add salt to food in the kitchen or at the dinner table. That brings the total average daily consumption of sodium to between 4100 and 6000 mg. The U.S. Food and Nutrition Board recommends that healthy adults consume only 1100 to 3300 mg of sodium per day.

The effect of excess sodium intake over a lifetime is strongly correlated with the development of high blood pressure. As much as 20 percent of the population will suffer high blood pressure if sodium consumption is too great. High blood pressure has three side effects: strokes, heart attacks, and kidney failure. Excess sodium can also lead to water retention and bloating. Because sodium binds water, it tends to interfere with the body's ability to properly regulate water balance. As if all this were not enough reason for cutting back on your salt intake, excess sodium is mildly toxic and caustic to body tissues.

Even though prepared and fast foods already contain a lot of sodium, one-fourth to one-third of your daily sodium intake is discretionary. If you cut down or eliminate the salt you add to food and cut back on high-sodium processed foods and beverages, you can keep your sodium intake within safe boundaries. At first you may find that unsalted foods taste a little flat. Don't worry; soon the nerve endings on your tongue will begin to transmit new and interesting tastes to your brain, and the real flavors of the food will emerge. Your taste buds will reawaken and, eventually, you'll find you no longer like salty foods.

If you find it difficult to give up the taste of salt, try a salt substitute. Most contain potassium in place of sodium. If you suffer from any form of kidney trouble, check with your doctor to make sure that additional potassium will not harm you.

Salt Content in Food

Foods that contain less than 25 mg of sodium:

- 12 oz. soda water
- 12 oz. diet soft drinks

Less than 75 mg of sodium:

- 3 oz. chicken
- 3 oz. turkey
- 3 oz. fresh fish
- 3 oz. canned tuna or salmon (low-sodium, water-packed)

Less than 120 mg of sodium:

- 1 cup low-fat milk
- 1 cup low-fat yogurt
- 1/2 cup cottage cheese
- 1/4 cup shellfish
- 3 oz. shrimp
- 3/4 cup lobster
- 3/4 cup oysters
- 2 oz. clams
- 1 slice bread
- 3 low-fat crackers

Less than 240 mg of sodium:

    1 oz. of most low-fat cheeses

    ½ cup of tomato juice

    2 tbsp. of prepared Italian dressing

    1 cup of most breakfast cereals

Less than 360 mg of sodium:

    1 oz. turkey or chicken breast cold cuts

    5 olives

Less than 1000 mg of sodium:

    2 tsp. baking powder

    1 bouillon cube

    1 dill pickle

    ½ tsp. table salt

    1 cup of canned or packaged soups

Sources of Fluids

Water—Water should be your most important source of fluids. Unfortunately, tap water is always an unknown quantity; you never really know how safe it is. The United States Environmental Protection Agency has found over 700 organic chemicals in drinking water. Forty of these have been shown to cause cancer in laboratory animals. Three—benzene, chloromethyl ether, and vinyl chloride—are associated with cancer in humans.

Make sure that your drinking water is safe. Installing a high-quality water purification system in your home is often a smart idea. Have your water tested by a laboratory if you have any doubts about its purity. If you use bottled water, select brands that have undergone distillation, reverse osmosis, or a combination of reverse osmosis and deionization.

Coffee—Coffee in large quantities (40 cups or more per week) has been linked to cancer of the pancreas and the bladder. It seems to inhibit the cells from correcting genetic mistakes. However, the evidence overwhelmingly indicates that having two cups of coffee or tea per day is not a risk factor for disease. Some of the oils in stronger coffee products, such as espresso and Turkish coffee, raise cholesterol levels to a mild degree. If you are going to drink coffee, have it black or with one percent or non-fat milk; the saturated fat in cream, milk, and non-dairy creamer will do you no good. Adding sugar will increase the chance of enlarging your fat mass if your body does not have an immediate need for additional carbohydrates.

If you are trying to cut down on caffeine, try water-treated decaffeinated coffee or, even better, hot water with lemon, non-caffeinated herbal teas, or coffee substitutes.

Tea—Tea is grown in some 30 countries and, next to water, is the most widely consumed beverage in the world. Although there is only one plant, camellia sinesis, tea is manufactured as black (78 percent), green (20 percent), or oolong (2 percent). Black tea is more popular in western countries and green tea is consumed primarily in Asian countries, North Africa, and the Middle East. Leaves intended for green tea are picked by the same method as those picked for black. Black tea is fermented; green tea is not.

Fermentation alters the chemical structure of the tea leaf, permitting principal flavor attributes to emerge. However, green tea offers a higher concentration of polyphenol antioxidants. Three cups usually contains about 300 to 400 mg of polyphenol antioxidants. This represents a significant intake of antioxidant nutrients.

Animal cancer research using green tea is very compelling. In animal studies green tea has been shown to increase the activities of antioxidant and detoxification enzymes in the lungs, liver, and small intestine. Laboratory studies have suggested that green tea polyphenols may inhibit cancer by blocking the formation of cancer-causing nitrosamines and suppressing the activation of carcinogens in lung, breast, colon, and melanoma cancer cells. Green tea extracts also block estrogen from attaching to estrogen receptors on breast cells, a function associated with decreasing breast cancer risk.

With respect to human studies, the best evidence exists for the prevention of stomach cancer and cancer of the esophagus. There is some indication that green tea consumption may reduce the risk of pancreatic cancer, colon cancer, and bladder cancer; however, more research is required.

Other studies reveal that green tea may have a mild effect on lowering LDL cholesterol, raising HDL cholesterol, and reducing the stickiness of blood platelets and protecting LDL cholesterol from free radical damage. All of these are associated with reduced risk of heart attack and stroke.

My view is that most of us would do well to substitute more green tea for coffee, black tea, and other herbal teas, as a daily beverage. To avoid the stimulant effects of the caffeine, decaffeinated green tea products are widely available.

Alcohol—Studies show that, although one to two alcoholic drinks per day may reduce your risk of heart disease, this amount of alcohol can also increase the risk of colon, breast, prostate, and other cancers. (One drink equals one beer, a five-ounce glass of wine, or one ounce of hard liquor.) The protective effects against heart disease arise from the ability of alcohol to raise HDL cholesterol levels and reduce the stickiness of blood platelets. It's been suggested too that alcohol reduces stress by its sedative effects and so is beneficial to the heart. However, aerobic exercise is a better way to raise your HDL levels and lower stress, and there are safer ways to reduce the stickiness of your blood.

Alcohol consumption accounts for at least three percent of all cancers, making it the second-most important lifestyle cause of cancer (after cigarette smoking, which is responsible for approximately 30 percent of all cancers). Alcohol is loaded with empty calories and is a classified as a co-carcinogen, in that it carries free radicals into the cells, allowing them to cause genetic damage. Smoking cigarettes contributes to cancers of the lungs, mouth, esophagus, stomach, bladder, pancreas, and kidney. If you smoke and drink at the same time, the alcohol acts as a co-carcinogen; your risk of developing mouth cancer increases 15 times compared to smoking without drinking. Alcohol speeds the delivery of free radicals to your genetic material, and it carries many impurities into the body that may indirectly increase your risk of cancer.

Alcohol consumption also is a leading cause of liver damage and liver cirrhosis, and is associated with many deaths and injuries each year from automobile accidents. Alcohol generates an enormous number of free radicals and thereby accelerates the aging process of our cells. One has only to examine the face of an alcoholic to see the pronounced aging effects of alcohol on the body. Finally, alcohol weakens your immune system.

In the long run, you will probably be healthier if you don't drink alcohol, or limit your consumption to no more than one drink in any 24-hour period. All indications suggest that our bodies can safely detoxify one alcoholic drink per day before we put ourselves at increased risk for cancer. Nonetheless, every alcoholic drink you consume generates free radicals and carries the potential to accelerate the aging process. If you are planning to slow the aging process and reduce your risk of chronic degenerative diseases, you must be very careful with alcohol consumption.

Juice—When you drink juice, it is best to dilute it first. Drink ¼ cup of unsweetened juice with ¾ cup of water. Pure juice has had much of its fiber stripped away, so the sugar in the juice, whether added or natural, will be digested too fast, resulting in a bombardment of glucose into your bloodstream.

Diet Soft Drinks and Soda Water—Most regular soft drinks contain white sugar, which can add empty refined carbohydrate calories to your diet, raising blood triglyceride levels and increasing your body fat. These drinks can also upset blood sugar levels by causing a sugar rush. If you like carbonated beverages, soda water or carbonated mineral water with lemon or lime are wiser choices. The occasional diet soft drink may be another alternative, but don't overdo it, as the jury is still out on the possible adverse effects of aspartame.

Aspartame was introduced to the market over two decades ago. Its presence in diet soft drinks, yogurt products, and many other prepared foods has been the focus of controversy ever since. Aspartame consists of two amino acids—aspartic acid and phenylalanine. The critics of aspartame claim that one of the by-products of aspartame metabolism in the body is formaldehyde, a well-known embalming agent. Rat studies show that high intakes of aspartame create what are known as formaldehyde adducts by binding to proteins and nucleic acids, including DNA nucleic acids, in liver cells, kidney cells, and certain blood cells. Hence there is potential for genetic damage that may lead to increased cancer risk in these tissues.

Alarms have been raised that the high phenylalanine load supplied by aspartame can also cause damage to brain cells, perhaps increasing the risk of seizures and brain cancer and aggravating the symptoms of Parkinson's disease. Contradictory animal and human studies have so far failed to substantiate or support these allegations conclusively. A recent study at the Washington University

Medical School suggested a correlation between the introduction of aspartame and a 10 percent increase in the incidence of solid brain tumors, but subsequent examination of the data disputed any relationship between the two; the incidence of brain tumors has actually declined in recent years.

Prior to 1997 there had been over 6500 anecdotal reports of adverse reactions to aspartame, mostly headaches, seizures, and behavioral and cognitive changes. None have been substantiated, although clinical studies are underway to determine the potential adverse effects of long-term use of this popular artificial sweetener.

On the positive side, aspartame has been shown to reduce high blood pressure in rats due to the conversion of phenylalanine into the amino acid tyrosine. A study on human subjects showed that the inclusion of aspartame-containing foods in a weight loss program (low-fat, low-calorie) resulted in an average reduction of 23 pounds in male participants and 16.5 pounds in female subjects. All participants reported feeling good and sleeping well, with no untoward side effects.

Aspartame's ability to form formaldehyde adducts within DNA is of some concern, yet the totality of evidence to date indicates that it is not increasing the risk of brain tumors or other cancers. Proponents of aspartame cite a study published in *Regulatory Toxicology and Pharmacology* in 2002, a respected scientific journal, which reviewed the safety profile of aspartame's twenty-year history in the market, as well as pre-market toxicology studies. The authors of this review concluded that the safety testing of aspartame has gone well beyond that required to evaluate the safety of a food additive, that aspartame is safe, and that there are no unresolved questions regarding its safety when used as intended. Even so, because research continues, my advice is to not overdo it with aspartame-containing foods and beverages, limiting your consumption to one or two servings per day (roughly 80 mg of aspartame).

Starting Right Now...

Pay attention to what you are drinking and how much. Increase the amount by one or two glasses a week until you are consuming six to eight glasses of fluids each day. You may include beverages such as decaffeinated coffee, tea, and soda. Do not count coffee or tea containing caffeine or alcohol: their fluid content is offset by the fact that they increase water loss through urination.

*For access to the references to Step 1 and additional education on wellness please visit the author's web site at **www.renaisante.com***

STEP 2

Reap the Benefits of Lifelong Supplements

Lifelong Supplement Number 1: High-potency Multivitamin and Mineral

As we learned in Step 1, a healthy diet is the primary source of the vitamins, minerals, and protective nutrients that will help prevent many degenerative conditions. However, to maximize your defenses against cancer, heart disease, and other degenerative diseases, and to slow the aging process, you also need supplements. It's estimated that sixty percent of North Americans take a daily vitamin/mineral supplement. Regular users cite these motivations:

- to enhance energy and well-being;
- to help defend against diseases such as cancer, heart disease, osteoporosis, and dementia;
- to help manage existing health conditions (e.g., arthritis; diabetes);
- to slow the aging process.

Some people still argue that we can derive all the vitamins and minerals we need from food alone. But do your homework on this subject, and you'll find that 80 to 90 percent of people don't reach their daily recommended allowances—or even come close. Results from the National Health and Nutrition Examination Surveys (both surveys 1 and 2) showed these results, which were a cross-sectional surveys of the American population. Marginal nutrient deficiencies are present in as many as 50 percent of non-users of supplement products. Furthermore, the daily allowance levels set by the government identify only the minimums required to guard against severe diseases (scurvy, pellagra, beriberi). They are not intended as guidelines for the optimal intake levels that help prevent degenerative diseases while maximizing our well-being and longevity.

As part of an overall wellness and anti-aging program, taking a high-potency multivitamin and mineral each day is crucial. Most multiple vitamin products contain all vitamins and minerals from vitamin A to zinc, but often at insufficient doses to provide the advantages you are seeking.

Free Radical Damage

It is widely accepted in the scientific community that free radicals cause cancer, accelerate aging, and contribute to the development and progression of heart disease and stroke, Alzheimer's disease and age-related cognitive decline, cataracts and macular degeneration of the eye, weakening of the immune system, skin cancer, wrinkles, and similar degenerative conditions. In fact, these harmful agents are believed to play a role in more than sixty different health conditions.

A free radical is a molecule with an unpaired electron. Electrons usually orbit the nucleus of an atom in pairs, one spinning clockwise and the other spinning counter-clockwise. A group of atoms makes up a molecule. A molecule with an unpaired electron will use the easiest means available to become whole and stable: it will strip an electron from a neighboring molecule that was otherwise minding its own business. The neighbour is now a free radical and must in turn steal an electron from another nearby molecule. This chain reaction of free radical formation is known to cause damage to cellular structures, including the cell's membrane, its enzymes, its DNA (its genetic blueprint) and its mitochondria (the energy-producing machinery of the cell). Studies show that free radical damage to the DNA of the cell can lead to cancer. Cigarette smoke, for example, is loaded with free radicals that attack the DNA of lung cells, creating cancerous mutations. It's estimated that cigarette smoke, including second-hand smoke, is responsible for approximately 30 percent of all human cancers.

There are many other sources of free radicals besides cigarette smoke. It may surprise you to learn that some of the oxygen we inhale is transformed into free radicals during the course of normal metabolism. These oxygen radicals likewise cause damage to body cells and tissues. When you cut open an apple and leave it exposed to the air for a few minutes, it turns brown. That is an oxygen free radical attack, and the same kind of reaction occurs in the body. Many researchers have demonstrated that this type of oxidizing over a lifetime is responsible for much of the aging of our tissues. In other words, we don't age, we actually slowly rot—just like the apple. Oxygen is a double-edged sword in that we need it to produce energy—without it we would die within three minutes or so—but at the same time, up to five percent percent of the oxygen in our cells is converted into very aggressive oxygen free radicals. In addition to cigarette smoke and oxygen, there are countless environmental and food-borne free radicals that can enter the body. Here are some harmful yet common examples:

- Alcohol—generates many free radicals and is responsible for approximately three percent percent of all human cancers in North America;
- Heterocyclic amines—found in barbecued, blackened, or Cajun-style meat or fish;

- Polycyclic aromatic hydrocarbons (PAH)—formed when the fat in meat drips onto the barbecue coals. The resulting smoke contains PAH, which infuses the food on the grill. Smoked meat and fish are known to contain high levels of PAH, and regular consumption of these foods is associated with an increased incidence of stomach and esophageal cancers;

- Pesticides such as DDT;

- Nitrosamines—formed when you consume foods like processed meats that contain nitrates and nitrite salts. Once in the intestinal tract, nitrates combine with protein amino acids to form cancer-causing nitrosamines;

- Ultraviolet light from the sun and tanning beds—UV light converts oxygen in skin cells into free radicals by injecting them with an unpaired electron from the photon energy in UV-light waves. These free radicals then go on to cause accelerated skin aging and increase the risk of skin cancer. UV light can also reach deep into the dermal layers and cause cross-linking of collagen fibers, which results in skin wrinkling.

- X-rays—radiation beams fired through the body initiate free radical formation in the our cells in much the same way that UV light initiates free radicals in skin cells;

- Air pollution—contains many free radicals, among them nitrous oxide and polycyclic aromatic hydrocarbons;

- Occupational free radicals—include substances such as carbon tetrachloride, asbestos, vinyl chloride, and heavy metals like mercury, cadmium, and lead.

Your body will come into contact with innumerable free radical insults over its lifetime. Reducing your exposure to free radicals as much as possible is important, but it is also vital to optimize your antioxidant defenses.

Antioxidants to the Rescue

Antioxidants have the ability to intercept, suppress, and neutralize free radicals, converting them into stable, non-harmful substances, and thus prevent or halt free radical damage to your tissues. Antioxidant molecules donate an electron or absorb an electron from a free radical molecule, without being converted into free radicals themselves. Fortunately, the body naturally produces several antioxidant enzymes such as glutathione peroxidase, catalase, and superoxide dismutase to help reduce free radical damage to the body. Without these enzymes to protect us from oxygen free radicals alone, we would all be dead within hours. They enable us to live in the earth's atmosphere of 21 percent oxygen, and to use oxygen to power energy production in our cells. However, these antioxidant enzymes require activation by certain minerals, among them manganese, magnesium, zinc, copper, and selenium. Our bodies also require additional protection from nutritional antioxidants such as vitamin A, vitamin C, vitamin E, beta-carotene, lycopene, lutein and zeaxantin, and bioflavonoids. Studies conducted over the past 25 years have produced evidence that supplementing with these nutritional antioxidants, at levels beyond what food alone can provide, can be significant in preventing degenerative diseases and in slowing the aging process.

Your lifelong wellness and anti-aging plan must include maximizing your defenses against free radical damage by consuming at least five servings of fruit and vegetables per day, and by acquiring the additional protection of a daily antioxidant-enriched, high-potency multivitamin and mineral supplement.

Antioxidants Reduce Cancer Risk

Research studies undertaken in the 1980s, in particular those by researchers in Finland and Switzerland, provided some of the first conclusive evidence that people who have higher intakes of vitamin C and beta-carotene, and who maintain appreciable blood levels of them through their lives, have a markedly lower risk of cancers than individuals with lower intakes or blood levels of these nutrients. Antioxidants like vitamin C, beta-carotene, vitamin E and others were shown to suppress free radicals that can cause cancerous mutations in cell DNA.

The *American Journal of Clinical Nutrition* reported in 1991 that a high total carotenoid intake (beta-carotene, lycopene, and lutein) had been linked with a significant reduction in the risk of cancers of the lung, stomach, breast, bladder, and colon a year later. A review published in Nutrition and Cancer reported on approximately 90 epidemiological studies that examined the role of vitamin C or vitamin C-rich foods in cancer prevention. According to those findings, the evidence was strong that vitamin C might protect against cancers of the esophagus, oral cavity, stomach, and pancreas and was substantial for cancers of the cervix, rectum, breast, and lung. As for vitamin E, the association between serum vitamin E levels and subsequent cancer risk was examined in at least 12 longitudinal studies. These found, on average, a three percent lower blood vitamin E level among individuals who later developed the disease. Vitamin E appeared to be especially protective against cancers of the stomach, pancreas, colon, and rectum, and, with selenium, of the reproductive organs in women. Since these early reports, much additional research has been undertaken to examine the relationship between antioxidants and cancer prevention even more closely.

Colon Cancer

As mentioned earlier, colon cancer is now the number two cause of cancer death in North America and colonoscopy testing is becoming routine for those over the age of fifty. A number of antioxidants have been identified as important to its repression.

Selenium is a trace mineral that is known to prevent chemically induced colon cancer in animal studies. In one study with rats that were fed a known cancer-causing chemical, the rats whose diets were supplemented with selenium had a tumor yield of only three percent, whereas the rats who received no selenium supplement had a 29 percent tumor yield. Other animal studies have shown that selenium supplements can reduce the incidence of intestinal tumors by fifty percent compared with animals given the cancer-causing agent without them.

Human observation studies are equally impressive. For example, areas in North America with low soil and crop selenium concentrations show higher incidences of colon and rectal cancers. In a study of U.S. veterans, blood levels of selenium were measured in subjects with and without colorectal cancer. Those with blood selenium levels below 128 micrograms per liter were 4.2 times more likely to have one or more cancerous polyps. In a separate clinical trial using selenium to reduce risk of skin cancer, 1312 subjects were given either 200 micrograms of selenium or a placebo daily for almost five years. Those taking the selenium experienced a 58 percent reduction in colon and rectal cancers compared to subjects taking the placebo.

More recently, in a study by Dr. Mark Russo and associates at the University of North Carolina (Chapel Hill), patients who were referred for a colonoscopy assessment were given blood tests as well. The researchers reported that the average blood level of selenium for patients with cancerous lesions was 107 micrograms per liter, compared to 120 micrograms per liter for the cancer-free subjects. An increase of 30 micrograms per liter in blood selenium level was associated with a 50 percent reduction in risk of colon cancer lesions.

The authors concluded that their data supported the protective effect of selenium against colon and rectal cancers after adjustments for factors as smoking, alcohol intake, use of dandruff shampoo (which contains selenium), and diet.

There are several ways that selenium is thought to reduce cancer risk. First, it may increase the levels of the naturally produced antioxidant enzyme glutathione peroxidase, a strong anti-cancer agent within the body. Selenium also decreases the formation of the cancer-permissive hormone known as prostaglandin series-2, which we last saw as a by-product of polyunsaturated fats in high-fat meat and dairy products. Finally, selenium metabolism itself may initiate the programmed death of cancer and precancerous cells.

The average person's intake of selenium from food sources is about 50 micrograms daily, not enough to maximize its anti-cancer defenses, according to the available research. Selenium consumed as a dietary supplement at 100 to 200 micrograms per day has been shown to reduce the incidence of lung, colorectal, and prostate cancer in humans. As reported by Dr. B. Combs and fellow researchers in 1996, selenium blood levels of approximately 120 mcg/ml (1.5 umol/ml) may be optimal for cancer prevention in general. The most recent estimates suggest that women require a minimum of 96 micrograms per day and men require at least 120 micrograms per day to support blood levels at 120 mcg/ml. Toxicity of selenium begins at doses of 1,000 micrograms per day, so 100-200 micrograms of selenium supplement from a multiple vitamin is extremely safe.

Vitamin E has also been shown to reduce the risk of colon cancer in many animal and human studies.

Like selenium, vitamin E inhibits the formation of the dangerous prostaglandin hormone series-2, which encourages the rapid division of tumor cells and helps cancer cells escape surveillance by the body's immune system. By suppressing the formation of prostaglandin series-2, vitamin E discourages tumor cell growth and enables the immune system to more effectively identify and destroy any cancer cells that may emerge.

Early studies dating back to 1982 demonstrated that 400 mg of vitamin E and 400 mg of vitamin C, when taken daily, dramatically reduced the formation of cancer-causing agents in the colons of test subjects.

More recently, the Iowa Women's Health Study demonstrated a very strong protective effect for vitamin E. This large-scale study of 35,000 women between 55 and 66 years of age tracked subjects who had no previous history of cancer. After four years, it produced convincing data that a high intake of vitamin E was associated with a reduced risk of colon cancer. Women in the top 20 percent level of vitamin E intake had a 66 percent lower chance of developing colon cancer than women ingesting vitamin E in the lowest 20 percent intake range. In almost all cases, those with a high intake were taking supplements containing vitamin E.

I recommend that adults ingest 400 I.U. of vitamin E per day from a high-potency multivitamin and mineral to help prevent colon and other cancers. Vitamin E is fat-soluble, so you must take it with a meal that provides some fat in order for it to be absorbed from your intestinal tract into the bloodstream. The same is true for vitamin A, beta-carotene, lycopene, lutein, vitamin D, and vitamin K.

In epidemiological and prospective studies and in intervention trials, vitamin C has been consistently linked to a reduced risk of colon cancer. It acts as an antioxidant in the intestinal tract and at sufficient levels will decrease the concentrations of cancer-causing chemicals in fecal matter. Vitamin C also blocks the formation of cancer-causing nitrosamines through the entire intestinal tract. In one two-and-a-half year study of colon polyps sufferers, it reduced the recurrence of colon polyps by 35 percent, compared to 23 percent in the placebo group.

Prostate Cancer

Prostate cancer is the most common cancer among men in North America. Studies suggest a link between oxygen free radicals and the development of tumors in the prostate, but it is also well known that proper diet and the use of supplements can reduce prostate cancer incidence.

The emerging research suggests that the antioxidant function of supplementary vitamin E, selenium and lycopene hold promise for its prevention. In the Alpha-Tocopherol, Beta-Carotene Cancer Prevention Study, reported in 1998 by Dr. O.P. Heinonen and colleagues, long-term supplementary doses of vitamin E were associated with a 32 percent decrease in the incidence of the disease. Over the eight-year period of the study, death from prostate cancer was 41 percent lower among men receiving the vitamin E supplement.

Examinations of blood levels in patients with prostate cancer have revealed low levels of selenium, with those at the lowest levels exhibiting as much as a 5.8 times higher risk of dying from the disease than those with the highest selenium levels. The correlation was supported by a four-and-a-half year study conducted by Dr. L. Clark and fellow researchers in 1996, in which the administration of selenium supplements was associated with a 63 percent lower incidence of prostate cancer.

The Health Professionals Follow-up Study of some 40,000 men aged 40 to 75 years of age also endorsed antioxidant benefits. The 1995 report linked a significant decrease in the risk of prostate cancer to higher intakes of lycopene, the most effective of the major carotenoids in destroying oxygen free radicals. An intake level of at least six mg per day was associated with a 21 percent reduction in prostate cancer incidence, compared with consuming less than 2.3 mg per day. It is estimated that a minimum four to six mg daily intake of lycopene is required for prostate protection.

Breast Cancer

Several epidemiological and clinical intervention studies have suggested that vitamin E supplementation can inhibit the development of breast cancer. The Nurses' Health Study, which has followed approximately 88,000 U.S. female nurses aged 34 to 59 years of age since 1980, found a 16 percent decreased risk of breast cancer in women within the top 20 percent range of vitamin E intake, compared to those in the lowest 20 percent range. Most women in the high range took vitamin E supplements in some form.

Vitamin E supplementation is also linked to a reduction in the spread and progression of breast cancer in women who already have the disease. According to a recent study by Dr. A. Fleischauer and others, breast cancer survivors taking vitamin E supplements experienced a 25 to 35 percent decrease in recurrence and mortality compared to non-users of vitamin E supplements. A cocktail of various antioxidants was shown to be helpful in a study by Dr. K. Lockwood and colleagues. They conducted an 18-month review of 32 women with breast cancer, all of whom were put on a nutritional protocol consisting of high-dose antioxidants and other nutrients. The women were between 32 and 81 years of age and classified as high-risk because their tumors had spread to the lymph nodes under the arm. The daily nutritional supplement, which was added to the normal surgical and therapeutic treatments for breast cancer, consisted of a combination of vitamin C, 2850 mg; vitamin E, 2500 IU; beta-carotene, 32.5 IU; selenium, 387 mcg; along with secondary vitamins and minerals, essential fatty acids (1.2 gm gamma linolenic acid and 3.5 gm omega-3 fatty acids), and coenzyme Q10 (90 to 390 mg per day). At the end of the study, none of the patients showed signs of further metastases, quality of life was improved (no weight loss, reduced use of painkillers) and six patients showed apparent partial remission. The results indicated that various antioxidants and other nutrients can work synergistically to help contain and prevent cancer.

Cervical Cancer

Antioxidants such as vitamin E, beta-carotene, and other carotenoids have been shown to protect against cervical cancer in certain studies. In some elevated blood levels of folic acid, beta-carotene, lycopene, and vitamin E were found effective against cervical dysplasia, a precancerous condition of the cervix. In a recent study of 32 women by Dr. P. Kanetsky and fellow researchers, it was found that women with higher intake and blood levels of lycopene were one-third as likely to have cervical dysplasia as those with the lowest one-third of lycopene blood levels. In addition, women who got more vitamin A were one-fourth as likely to develop dysplasia as women with the lowest one-third of vitamin A blood levels.

In another study of patients with mild or moderate cervical dysplasia, 30 subjects were treated with 30 mg (50,000 I.U.) of beta-carotene orally every day. More than 70 percent of patients showed a reversal of their condition after six months. The evidence is persuasive that nutrition and antioxidant supplementation can play a vital role in the prevention of cervical dysplasia and, in some cases, can reverse this condition in its early and moderate stages.

Stomach Cancer

Like colon cancer, stomach cancer is closely linked to nitrosamines, a known group of environmental carcinogens. On average, North Americans consume approximately 74 mg of nitrates per day, thanks to processed meats, alcoholic beverages, and plant foods grown in soils treated with nitrogen fertilizers. Both vitamin C and vitamin E can block the formation of nitrosamines in the stomach and intestinal tract when taken as supplements with, or shortly after, a meal containing nitrates and protein. Taking 500 mg of vitamin C twice a day has been shown to block as much as 85 to 100 percent of nitrosamine formation under conditions of a high nitrate intake. Vitamin E has demonstrated similar effects: a daily dosage of 400 IU can help prevent the formation of nitrosamines.

Antioxidants Reduce Heart Disease Risk

The substantial body of evidence that vitamin E and vitamin C supplementation can reduce the risk of heart disease and other cardiovascular conditions maybe truly life-saving. Cardiovascular disease accounts for nearly 50 percent of all deaths in North America.

In 1987 Dr. F. Gey and his colleagues published the results of an extensive European study in which researchers collected blood samples from healthy men who lived in areas with high heart disease mortality (southwest Finland, north Karelia), medium mortality (Northern Ireland) and low mortality (Switzerland and southern Italy). The average blood vitamin E levels were found to be significantly higher in regions with low heart disease mortality, compared with those in regions with higher rates. In a subsequent, more detailed study of 16 regions in 10 European countries, the MONICA study is a weird type of an acronym for Multinational MONItoring of trends and determinants in CArdiovascular disease. It began in the early 1980's assessing overall trends in 21 countries for cardiovascular disease risk, over a 10 year period. It followed 10 million men and women age 25-64 during the study period. It is one of the largest cardiovascular disease studies performed to date. Researchers again reported a strong relationship between high blood vitamin E levels and low rates of heart disease mortality. This relationship has been borne out by the research of other investigators who have studied angina patients in the United States, cardiovascular disease mortality in the Netherlands, and heart disease rates in Finland.

In the Nurses' Health Study, women who were free from cardiovascular disease and cancer at the beginning of the study showed a 41 percent reduction in risk of heart disease among those who consumed daily vitamin E supplements (greater than or equal to 100 I.U.) for at least two years, compared with those who did not, after eight years of follow up. This finding held true even after factoring in other heart disease risk factors. In this same study, the risk of ischemic stroke was also reduced by 29 percent in nurses using vitamin E supplementation at or above 100 I.U. per day.

Similar results were seen in men in the Health Professionals Follow-up Study. It enlisted 39,910 men aged 40 to 75 years old in 1986 who were free of cardiovascular disease, diabetes, or high cholesterol at the beginning of the study. Those taking vitamin E supplements showed the greatest reduction in risk of heart disease (a 46 percent reduction) compared with non-supplement users. The protective dosage was found to be 100 to 350 I.U. per day in this study. As with the Nurses' Health Study, vitamin E supplementation below 100 I.U. per day did not provide significant protection against heart disease.

In the mid-nineties Dr. H.N. Hodis and fellow researchers measured the progression of coronary artery narrowing, or atherosclerosis, in 162 nonsmoking men aged 40 to 59. Those men who took vitamin E supplements experienced a significant slowdown in the narrowing of their arteries compared with non-supplement users. The apparent benefit once again affected only those taking more than 100 I.U. of vitamin E daily. In this study subjects who received cholesterol-lowering medication in addition to vitamin E supplements showed actual regression in coronary artery narrowing. The ability to reverse heart disease by this form of combination therapy is a truly remarkable finding.

Other intervention trials using vitamin E supplements have demonstrated their beneficial effects in combating atherosclerosis elsewhere in the body and in the recovery of coronary angioplasty patients. Overall, studies indicate that daily vitamin E supplementation exceeding 100 IU is associated with a 40 percent reduction in risk for heart attack and other cardiovascular problems related to atherosclerosis.

Vitamin E appears to protect against cardiovascular disease in three ways. First, as an antioxidant it travels in the bloodstream bound to LDL cholesterol. As part of this cholesterol complex, it intercepts free radicals that might otherwise damage cholesterol and its related unsaturated fats. Cholesterol damaged by free radicals is much more likely to adhere to artery walls as plaque. Second, vitamin E regulates the rate at which smooth muscle within the artery wall will grow and proliferate. Like plaque build-up, this process can also contribute to a harmful narrowing of the arteries.

The third protective action of vitamin E is its ability to reduce the stickiness of blood platelets. Platelets are the blood cells that clump together and form clots. They prevent us from bleeding to death every time we nick ourselves with a sharp object or develop a nosebleed. However, several common lifestyle factors (smoking, lack of exercise, and a diet high in unsaturated fats) encourage platelets to be excessively sticky and to form abnormal and potentially fatal clots or mini-plugs inside the arteries. Ideally, platelets should clump together to save your life, not to end it. Vitamin E regulates platelet stickness and discourages the abnormal clumping that could obstruct blood flow.

As demonstrated by a number of prominent researchers, blood levels of vitamin E necessary to materially reduce free radical attack of LDL cholesterol, to inhibit smooth muscle growth in the arteries, and to reduce platelet stickiness are achieved only through supplementation. At least 100 I.U. of vitamin E per day are required to obtain a cardio-protective effect. In my view, a daily dosage of 400 I.U. is ideal for the purpose of prevention and anti-aging.

What about vitamin C and heart disease? In the Monica Study previously mentioned, scientists demonstrated that vitamin C blood levels above 50 micromoles per litre were associated with more than a 50 percent reduction in heart disease mortality rates. Low blood levels of both vitamin C and vitamin E were stronger predictors of future heart disease mortality than were high blood cholesterol levels, smoking or high blood pressure, which are known cardinal risk factors.

In a 20-year follow-up study of a group of patients in the United Kingdom over 65 years of age, low vitamin C status was strongly associated with increased risk of death from stroke. A Swiss study reported on in 1993 uncovered an identical finding on related research by Dr. D. Harats, published in 1998, showed that subjects ingesting 500 mg per day of vitamin C exhibited decreased free radical damage to cholesterol.

A number of studies have demonstrated that vitamin E protects blood cholesterol from free radical attack. It appears that vitamin C shares this important role as a water-soluble antioxidant circulating in the bloodstream. In fact, high doses of vitamin C (500-1,000 mg daily) have lowered blood cholesterol in high cholesterol patients receiving supplementation. But research in Finland suggested an interesting relationship between vitamins E and C and the risk of heart attack. Dr. R. Salonen found that low vitamin E status (from diet) was associated with increased risk only if vitamin C status was also low. Because vitamin C is required to regenerate vitamin E, this finding could explain the lack of protective effect of vitamin E alone. The two appear to work together to help protect us against heart attack, stroke, and other vascular diseases.

The recommended daily allowance for vitamin C is 60 mg. This nominal amount is insufficient to raise blood levels into a more protective range, discouraging free radical damage to blood cholesterol and helping to lower the total amount of cholesterol in the bloodstream. Alarmingly, 20 to 30 percent of U.S. adults fail to attain 60 mg of vitamin C each day from their diets. Ingesting at least 1000 mg of vitamin C per day, in two 500 mg doses, is the amount I recommend for general prevention and anti-aging.

Antioxidants Reduce Alzheimer's Disease and Dementia Risk

At any given moment, the brain is using at least 10 percent of the body's oxygen, thereby exposing the brain cells to significant levels of oxygen free radicals. Over a lifetime these free radicals can cause enough corrosive damage—much the way oxygen in the air can rust out a car—to interfere with the cells' normal function and ultimately to contribute to cell death. Researchers have shown that many brain and nerve degenerative diseases, including Alzheimer's disease and age-related cognitive decline or senile dementia, are strongly linked to free radical damage. At the same time, evidence is accumulating that individuals who take antioxidant supplements at protective dosages have a much lower risk of developing these conditions as they age.

In the Chicago Health in Aging Project, where 6000 people aged 62 to 102 were followed for three years, the average annual decline in cognitive score was 34 percent less in those with the highest vitamin E intake compared with those in the lowest intake group. A weak association was also established for vitamin C. In 1998 Dr M.C. Morris and his colleagues reported that among a group of 633 individuals 65 years and older, none of the vitamin E or vitamin C supplement users developed Alzheimer's disease during the 4.3 year follow-up study to the Chicago project.

In the Alzheimer's Disease Co-operative Study, Alzheimer's patients with moderately advanced disease were treated with 2,000 I.U. vitamin E a day or with a placebo. The results indicated that vitamin E supplementation was able to slow the functional deterioration of the brain significantly in these patients, delaying the need for nursing home placement and retarding the progression of the disease. Laboratory research results published in 1999 revealed that vitamin E inhibits free radical damage to brain cells induced by the Abeta-amyloid protein, a hallmark feature of Alzheimer's disease.

Meanwhile, other studies have shown that supplementation with vitamin E is effective in slowing the progression of Parkinson's disease and helps to control tardive dyskinesia, a condition involving involuntary repetitive movements of the face and head brought on by certain drugs that affect brain function.

Antioxidants Reduce Eye Disease Risk

The leading cause of blindness in people over the age of 55 in North America is age-related macular degeneration (AMD). Though the underlying causes are not fully understood, the evidence linking free radical damage to the development of AMD is strong and consistent. In daylight, ultraviolet light from the sun travels through the pupil to the back of the eye, where waves in the visible light spectrum stimulate the optic nerve, enabling vision to occur. However, the ultraviolet light at the back of the eye also induces free radical damage, which in turn can lead to macular degeneration. Along with the effects of ultraviolet light, smoking, atherosclerosis, and high blood pressure can contribute to the development of AMD.

Preliminary studies in humans backed up the evidence of earlier animal research that high blood levels of antioxidant vitamins and minerals could reduce the risk of AMD. One investigation revealed that individuals in the top 20 percent blood levels of selenium, vitamin C, and vitamin E had a 70 percent lower risk of developing AMD than did those with blood levels in the lowest 20 percent. In the Physicians' Health Study, male doctors taking vitamin E supplements had a 13 percent reduced risk of AMD.

Dietary intake of lutein and zeaxanthin (mostly dark green vegetables) plus supplementation with these two carotenoids has been shown to increase the amount of macular pigment in the back of the eye. That acts as a shield, protecting the optic nerve from free radical assault. In fact the area around the optic nerve is known as the macula lutea, due to its high concentration of lutein.

One study showed that adults with the highest intake of lutein had a 57 percent reduced risk of developing AMD compared to those with low levels of this carotenoid.

The most convincing evidence that antioxidant supplements provide protection against AMD was published in 2001 by researchers of the Age-Related Eye Disease Study, a multi-center, intervention trial involving 4,757 patients between the ages of 55 and 80 years old. In this study, conducted by the U.S.-based National Eye Institute, patients who were at high risk of developing more advanced stages of AMD reduced their risk by approximately 25 percent when treated with a high-dose combination of vitamin C, vitamin E, beta-carotene, and zinc. According to the NEI, antioxidant supplementation is the first effective treatment ever shown to successfully slow the progression of the disease. Participants in this double-blind, placebo-controlled clinical study, who suffered from varying degrees of AMD, were given one of four treatments. The best results occurred in those taking both antioxidant and zinc supplements in these doses:

- vitamin C – 500 mg;
- vitamin E – 400 IU;
- beta-carotene – 25,000 IU;
- zinc – 80 mg.

Antioxidant supplements have also been shown to prevent cataracts (white, opaque lesions that form on the normally transparent lens of the eye). They occur as a result of damage to the protein structure of the lens. Strong evidence exists that free radical damage from ultraviolet light and radiation exposure contribute to later-life cataract development. The lens of the eye is devoid of the naturally-produced antioxidant enzymes, superoxide dismutase, catalase and glutathione peroxidase, and is completely dependent on nutritional antioxidants such as vitamin E, vitamin C, selenium, and carotenes for its antioxidant defenses.

Cataracts are the leading cause of all blindness and impaired vision in the United States. Forty thousand Americans are blind due to cataracts, and cataract surgery is the most prevalent major surgery among Medicare recipients in the U.S. A Canadian study by J. Robertson and fellow researchers suggested that if all Canadians over 55 years of age took an appropriate supplement of vitamin C and vitamin E every day, cataract incidence would be reduced by at least 50 percent and cut related health care costs in half. A number of intervention trials have demonstrated that 1000 mg of vitamin C per day can halt or slow the development of cataracts in the early stages. Other case-control and prospective studies have likewise linked higher blood levels and/or intake levels of vitamin C and vitamin E with a significant reduction in the risk of cataracts.

Antioxidants Slow Skin Wrinkling and Reduce Skin Cancer Risk

Premature aging of the skin and genetic damage to skin cells most commonly results from free radical damage induced by exposure to ultraviolet light from the sun and from tanning beds. This damage hastens the process of skin aging and wrinkling and creates cell mutations that lead to the development of skin cancers (basal cell carcinoma, squamous cell carcinoma, and melanoma). Avoiding overexposure to sunlight and other known sources of free radicals, wearing protective clothing, and using antioxidant-containing sun block products are all prudent strategies to minimize environmental skin injury.

The use of antioxidant supplements is another defense against free radical damage premature wrinkling and cancerous mutations. A 1998 double-blind, placebo-controlled study of human subjects demonstrated that those taking the vitamin C (2000 mg per day) and vitamin E (1000 I.U.) supplements had significantly less damage to their skin after UV-light exposure than did the group not given the supplement regime. They also showed considerably less sunburn reaction.

Investigation in this area strongly suggests that daily supplements of vitamins A, C, E, beta-carotene, selenium, and zinc, at levels above those typically consumed from food alone, provides the skin with additional and possibly essential antioxidant defenses to help slow skin aging and lend support to other skin cancer prevention initiatives.

Antioxidants Strengthen Your Immune System

Over the years, the immune system tends to become weaker and less efficient at combating germs that can cause serious infections and at identifying and destroying emerging cancer cells. Yet it is essential to maintain a strong, efficient immune system throughout your lifetime. Antioxidants can help maintain more optimal immune function as we age, and help to strengthen the immune system in individuals who are in an immune-compromised state.

Beta-carotene supplements, along with other carotenoids, have increased immune cell numbers and activity in animal and human tests. Placebo-controlled studies have shown their positive benefits in increasing the count of some white blood cells and enhancing cancer-fighting immune functions in healthy people consuming 25,000 to 100,000 IU per day. In double-blind trials in elderly subjects, 40,000 to 150,000 IU per day increased the effectiveness of immune cells that identify and kill emerging cancer cells. Supplementation at these high levels may be important to individuals who have already encountered cancer or whose immune systems are severely weakened by such diseases as hepatitis or HIV infection.

Vitamin C has been shown to stimulate the immune system by both elevating interferon levels and enhancing the activity of certain immune cells. A combination of vitamin A, vitamin C, and vitamin E significantly improved immune cell number and activity, compared to a placebo, in a group of hospitalized elderly patients. In another study involving human subjects, daily intake of a 1000 mg vitamin C plus 200 IU vitamin E for four months improved several measures of immune function.

Vitamin E supplementation has improved some aspects of immune-cell activity in the elderly. The effect is more pronounced with 200 IU per day, compared to lower doses (60 IU per day), according to double-blind research, according to studies performed in 1997 by S.N. Meydani, M. Meydani, and J.B. Blumberg as well as a second study by F.G. DeWaart and fellow researchers.

B Vitamins Also Prevent Cancer, Heart Disease and Dementia

In addition to antioxidants, a well-formulated high-potency multi-vitamin and mineral should include a B-50 complex comprising 50 mg of most of the B vitamins plus 400 mcg of folic acid, 50 mcg of vitamin B12, and 300 mcg of biotin. High B vitamin levels reduce risk of heart disease and certain inflammatory states, improve detoxification processes, and maintain brain and cognitive function. B vitamins are also essential for the synthesis of red blood cells and normal cell replication, and they are known for their anti-stress and anti-fatigue properties.

B Vitamins Reduce Risk of Cervical and Colon Cancer

Folic acid and vitamin B12 are essential to the body's production of the amino acid S-adenosylmethionine, one of the necessary building blocks of DNA. If folic acid and vitamin B12 levels fall, the amount of S-adenosylmethionine will decline, inhibiting the replication of healthy DNA cells from one generation to the next. Genetic errors will become more common and genetic linkages more fragile, prone to breakage or mutation. These alterations to genetic structure allow cancers to take hold in our DNA.

Women who are marginally deficient in folic acid are vulnerable to cervical dysplasia and cervical cancer. Apart from its role in DNA synthesis and repair, folic acid inhibits the ability of the human papillomavirus (HPV) to invade the DNA of surface cervical cells. Women who have experienced multiple sex partners are most likely to contract HPV, as contact with semen is the way cervical cells are typically exposed to the virus.

HPV is strongly associated with cervical cancer, and thus folic acid supplementation is important to help prevent its infection of cervical tissue.

Oral contraceptives are known to increase the rate of cell division of cervical cells, adding to the risk of cervical dysplasia. A number of studies have demonstrated that folic acid supplementation can reverse cervical megaloblastic changes and dysplasia, in patients using oral contraceptives. In one conducted by Dr. C.E. Butterworth and others, patients with mild and moderate degrees of cervical dysplasia showed reversal of their condition over a three-month trial period.

Childbearing women have been advised to ingest at least 400 mcg of folic acid daily to reduce the risk of spinal birth defects in their offspring. This same dosage appears to be effective in reducing the risk of cervical dysplasia as well.

With respect to colon cancer, Dr. E. Giovannucci and fellow researchers assessed the dietary habits of women in the Nurses' Health Study and men in the Health Professionals Follow-up Study for a period of one year. Of their 25,474 subjects, 895 developed polyps of the colon or rectum. A major finding was that high folic acid intake protected subjects against colorectal cancer. Women in the top 20 percent intake level of folic acid demonstrated a 34 percent decreased risk of colorectal cancer compared with those in the bottom 20 percent intake level. Among men, a 37 percent reduction in risk was observed for the highest 20 percent intake of folic acid versus the lowest 20 percent intake group. Users of multiple vitamins exhibited the greatest reduction in risk of colorectal cancer in this study and much of their protective effect was due to folic acid. Here too, 400 mcg per day is the dosage recommended.

B Vitamins and the Prevention of Heart Disease and Stroke

Just as folic acid and vitamin B12 are required for the production of essential compounds like S-adenosylmethionine in the body, so too are they necessary for the elimination of other naturally-produced agents that are not so desirable. Researchers have identified homocysteine, an amino acid that is formed in the course of normal metabolism, as a having a toxic effect on the cells that line our blood vessels. It increases the tendency of blood platelets to clump in the bloodstream and it stimulates the growth of muscle fibres into the arteries, both of which can impair blood flow. High blood levels of homocysteine signal an increased risk of cardiovascular, cerebrovascular (narrowed arteries in the brain) and peripheral vascular (narrowed arteries in the arms, hands, legs, and feet) disease. Ten percent of all heart attacks in the United States are attributed to elevated blood levels of homocysteine.

An appropriate intake of folic acid and vitamins B6 and B12 has been shown to reduce high homocysteine counts. In a 14-year follow-up of women in the Nurses' Health Study, subjects who took daily doses of folic acid and vitamin B6 above the recommended dietary allowances experienced a 45 percent reduced risk of fatal and non-fatal heart attacks. Findings from the Health Professionals Follow-up Study among male health practitioners likewise demonstrated a correlation between high folic acid intake and a significant reduction in heart disease risk. Many experts now recommend that the daily dietary allowance of folic acid be set at 400 mcg, a level most easily achieved through multivitamin and mineral supplements.

B Vitamins Preserve Memory and Cognitive Function

Deterioration of mental capacity has long been accepted as a condition of the normal aging process. In recent years, however, scientific evidence has demonstrated that certain natural health products and supplements are effective in preventing, reversing, or better managing cognitive impairment in older individuals. The Boston Veterans Affairs Normative Aging Study is one of many studies that have investigated the influence of nutrition on age-related disorders. Its results, published in 1996 in *The American Journal of Clinical Nutrition*, indicated that older individuals with low blood concentrations of vitamin B12, vitamin B6, and folic acid had the poorest scores of brain function as measured by a battery of cognitive tests.

In earlier studies clinical deficiencies of B vitamins have been implicated in a range of brain-related disorders, among them reversible dementia and electrophysiological dysfunction, including convulsions. In healthy older adults blood levels of B vitamins usually considered to be in the normal range were associated with poorer scores on tests of delayed recall, abstract reasoning, and selective attention. There is also good evidence that deficiencies of vitamin B12, folic acid, and vitamin B6 commonly increase with age.

B vitamins are known to be critical to brain chemistry and physiology. Vitamin B6 is a cofactor in the production of dopamine, norepinephrine, serotonin, and other chemical neurotransmitters. Vitamin B12 and folic acid are also required the synthesis of serotonin, adrenaline and norepinephrine. As described earlier, they are necessary for the production of S-adenosylmethionine, which has known anti-depressant properties. Vitamin B12 deficiency can result in de-insulation of nerve fibers, which will produce a constellation of neurological symptoms. Low intakes of B vitamins generally can lead to higher blood levels of homocysteine and narrowed arteries in the brain can cause serious cognitive dysfunction. In the Normative Aging Study, subjects with high levels of homocysteine performed like patients with mild Alzheimer's disease in tests measuring psychomotor speed.

There is growing support for the premise that optimal vitamin B levels can prevent, slow, or reverse the deterioration of memory and other mental capacities in older individuals. A 1992 double-blind study showed that daily supplementation with 20 mg of vitamin B6 (pyridoxine) improved memory performance in a group of men aged 70 to 79 years. Another study that same year by researchers Dr. D.C. Martin and associates showed that the administration of vitamin B12 to elderly individuals caused a "striking improvement" in various aspects of cognitive function.

B vitamins are crucial to the development and preservation of mental skills throughout our lifetimes. The sad reality is that many midlife and older members of society have poor dietary intake and nutritional status of the various B vitamins.

Bone Support Nutrients From a High-potency Multivitamin and Mineral

In North America, at least one in four women develops osteoporosis by age 50 and one in eight men develop the condition after age 50. In women, complications of osteoporotic fractures cause more deaths each year than breast and ovarian cancers combined. Preventing osteoporosis requires a lifelong strategy that includes an adequate daily intake of calcium, vitamin D, magnesium, copper, and zinc, which together are the essential bone-strengthening nutrients. Studies show that across the population most adolescents and adults fall short of their calcium requirements by 500 mg, on average, that is required to prevent future development of osteoporosis. Intakes of vitamin D, for calcium absorption, and zinc are also below the levels recommended by nutrition experts. Thus, a well-designed multiple vitamin, containing 500 mg of elemental calcium, 400 IU of vitamin D, 15 mg of zinc, 200 mg of magnesium, and 2 mg of copper, is an important lifelong strategy to help prevent osteoporosis.

The Benefits of a High-potency Multivitamin and Mineral Supplement

The truth is that it is impossible to acquire the optimal doses of every vitamin and mineral from food alone. In order to prevent degenerative diseases, maximize your health and wellbeing, and slow the aging process, it is absolutely necessary to take a high-potency multivitamin and mineral every day. By this I mean a multivitamin and mineral supplement that is antioxidant-enriched, contains a B-50 complex, and offers the proper doses of bone-building nutrients. This formula can not only help defend your body and mind against degenerative conditions, but it will enhance the texture of your skin, hair, and nails; improve sleep quality; strengthen your immune system; and boost your energy level.

Here is the high-potency multivitamin and mineral formulation I developed and recommend to my patients and other health practitioners:

Multivitamin & Mineral Daily Supplement

Water-soluble substances such as vitamin C are generally not stored well by the body, and it is best to replenish blood and tissue levels of water-soluble vitamins and minerals by taking supplements containing these nutrients twice daily, allowing 4-6 hours between intakes. These values represent the total daily levels from supplementation, but should be taken in two divided doses — at two separate meals.

(Continued)

(Continued)

Beta carotene	10,000 I.U.	Niacin	50 mg
Biotin	300 mcg	Pantothenic Acid	50 mg
Calcium	500 mg	Selenium	100 mcg
Chromium	50 mcg	Vitamin A	2500 I.U.
Citrus Bioflavonoids	50 mg	Vitamin B-1	50 mg
Copper	2 mg	Vitamin B-2	50 mg
Folic Acid	400 mcg	Vitamin B-6	50 mg
Iron	6 mg	Vitamin B-12	50 mcg
Lutein – 5%	6 mg	Vitamin C	1000 mg
Lycopene – %	6 mg	Vitamin D	400 I.U.
Magnesium	200 mg	Vitamin E (all-natural)	400 I.U.
Manganese	5 mg	Zinc	15 mg
Molybdenum	50 mcg		

Lifelong Supplement Number 2: Essential Fatty Acids

Essential fatty acids are the second supplement in your lifelong daily regimen. They play a vital role in the prevention of cancer and heart disease, help reduce and prevent inflammatory conditions such as arthritis, Crohn's disease, ulcerative colitis, eczema, and psoriasis; improve the softness and smoothness of your skin; and provide many other health benefits.

Essential fatty acids are important components of the outer skin or membrane of every cell. The membrane determines which chemicals and nutrients will be allowed to enter and exit the cell; essential fats influence the health of every cell in the body through their support of the structure and function of the cell membrane. In nerve cell membranes, for example, essential fatty acids facilitate nerve conduction, which enables the brain to think and to transmit impulses to other nerves, muscles, and organs. Within the cell membrane essential fatty acids are continually activated and converted into prostaglandin hormones, a process that allows essential fatty acids to supply their disease prevention and anti-aging effects to a wide range of tissues within the body. Not all prostaglandin hormones are so beneficial, however.

Prostaglandin Series-2 (PG-2) Causes Many Health Problems

There are three main types of prostaglandin hormones (PG): PG-1, PG-2, and PG-3. PG-1 and PG-3 have positive impacts on our health, while PG-2 can lead to highly undesirable effects. It encourages blood vessels to constrict and blood platelets to clot abnormally, thereby increasing the chance of heart attack, ischemic stroke, and high blood pressure. It also encourages inflammation, worsening arthritis and other joint, muscle and tendon conditions, including Crohn's disease and colitis. As described earlier, PG-2 is associated with greater risk of cancer in that it prompts rapid cell division. Finally, it can make the skin dry, rough, and scaly, and aggravate a number of common skin disorders, such as eczema, psoriasis, and possibly roscacea.

PG-2 is formed from an unsaturated fat known as arachidonic acid, found in high-fat meats and high-fat dairy products. As well, the over-consumption of linoleic acid, an unsaturated fat found in corn oil, sunflower seed oil, safflower seed oil, and mixed vegetable oils, promotes the production of arachidonic acid by the body. Higher cell membrane concentrations of arachidonic acid favor the synthesis of PG-2, contributing to a raft of health ills. Unfortunately, the typical North American diet is a rich source of arachidonic acid and linoleic acid, and most individuals produce too much PG-2.

You can lower your tissue concentrations of arachidoninc acid by choosing chicken, turkey or fish, instead of high-fat meat products, and non-fat or 1 percent milk and yogurt products. Exclude from your diet any cheese that is more than 3 percent milk fat, and use olive oil or canola oil in place of other vegetable oils in salad dressings. It's worth repeating that peanut oil may be used for stir-fries, but no oil can be safely used for deep-frying, which should be avoided. Olive oil and canola oil are good sources of monounsaturated fat, which does not participate in the formation of prostaglandin hormones and is known to help reduce cholesterol and contribute to cardiovascular health in other ways.

Supplement with Healthy Essential Fatty Acids That Make PG-1 and PG-3

The appropriate dietary changes will help prevent the formation of PG-2 but it is equally important to supplement your diet with the essential fatty acids that encourage the production of PG-1 and PG-3. These essential fatty acids promote good health by suppressing inflammation, dilating blood vessels, maintaining normal blood clotting, slowing the rate of cell division, and improving the smoothness and softness of the skin while healing various skin conditions.

The key building block for PG-1 is an unsaturated fat known as gamma-linolenic acid (GLA), which is found in high concentrations in borage oil (22 percent yield, compared to the better-known evening primrose oil, at 9 percent yield). GLA can also be formed in the body from linoleic acid, but individuals who suffer diabetes, eczema, or premenstrual syndrome have a defective enzyme that prevents the conversion of linoleic acid to GLA. The consumption of alcohol, refined sugars, and hydrogenated fats tends to inhibit this conversion, as does the aging process itself. Consequently virtually everyone has suboptimal cell membrane concentrations of GLA.

The solution is to take a borage oil supplement (22 percent GLA) every day to ensure high production of PG-1 hormones. Studies have shown that supplementation with GLA-containing oils can reduce pain and swelling in arthritis, including rheumatoid arthritis, and improve fibrocystic breast disease, PMS, and skin lesions, such as eczema. Even if you don't experience these conditions, it is still important to boost your synthesis of PG-1 with borage seed oil.

PG-3 is formed from an omega-3 unsaturated fat called eicos-apentaenoic acid (EPA), which is found in cold-water marine fish such as salmon, mackerel, anchovies, sardines, and tuna. The body can also convert the omega-3 fat alpha-linolenic acid (ALA) found in flaxseed oil (58 percent yield) into EPA, increasing the production of PG-3. Fish oil contains docosahexaenoic acid (DHA), another oil that the body can convert into EPA and thence, PG-3, if required. DHA enhances immune function and the development and function of the brain, and is essential to good vision.

PG-3 is considered very important for total body wellness, as it reduces risk of heart attacks by dilating blood vessels and discouraging abnormal blood clotting. It slows the rate of cell division and so reduces the risk, especially of breast, prostate, and colon cancer. PG-3 is also known to reduce inflammation, including skin inflammatory responses, a role it shares with PG-1.

Most individuals suffer unknowingly from an essential fatty acid deficiency or imbalance, thanks to modern agricultural and food processing methods and the typical North American diet. Neglecting these deficiencies can contribute to numerous health disorders, from cancer and heart disease to complexion problems, skin disorders, and inflammatory conditions. To ensure optimal essential fatty acid nutritional status, I recommend you take an essential fatty acid supplement that contains omega 3, 6, and 9 fatty acids, derived from equal amounts (400 mg each) of non-genetically modified flaxseed oil, borage oil, and a high yield fish oil (30 percent EPA/20 percent DHA) every day. For general health maintenance, I suggest two to three 1200 mg capsules daily. This simple practice can result in significant benefits for your health, your appearance, the rate at which your body will age, and your risk of future illness.

Essential Fatty Acid Daily Supplement

Each capsule should contain these ingredients and dosages, and individuals should consume 2-3 capsules per day for general health-promotion and anti-aging purposes. They can be taken all at once if that is most convenient or at intervals through the day. Essential fatty acids are fat-soluble and can be easily stored for later use by the body.

Essential Fatty Acid Source	Distinguishing Features	Amount
Borage Seed Oil modified seeds	Non-genetically	400 mg
Flaxseed Oil modified seeds	Non-genetically	400 mg
Fish Oil and 20 percent DHA	30 percent EPA	400 mg

Vitamins and Minerals as Co-Factors for PG-1 and PG-3 Synthesis

One final note: certain vitamins and minerals are required as co-factors in the enzymatic reactions that allow the cells of your body to convert healthy essential fatty acids into PG-1 and PG-3. For example, the conversion of ALA to EPA requires high levels of vitamin B6, zinc, magnesium, and niacin (vitamin B3). The synthesis of PG-1 and PG-3 requires the optimal intake of vitamin C, vitamin E, and selenium. Thus, in addition to all the advantages described earlier, the use of a high-potency multivitamin and mineral is also vital to the production of health-promoting prostaglandins.

Lifelong Supplement Number 3: Flaxseed Powder

One of the most versatile natural agents for the promotion of health and wellbeing among both men and women is ground flaxseed. Flaxseeds are an extremely rich source of secoisolariciresinol diglycoside (SLD); in fact, flaxseeds contain 800 times more SLD and related compounds than any other common food. Ingesting the equivalent of two heaping tablespoons, or approximately 45 to 50 gm of ground flaxseed (sometimes marketed as flaxseed powder) per day, helps support the health of the female reproductive organs and the male prostate gland. This level of daily intake will also lower blood cholesterol levels, enhance liver and gallbladder function, improve large bowel health, reverse fibrocystic breast disease, help support bone density by slowing calcium resorption, and improve the texture of the skin.

Flaxseed and Reproductive Organs

After ingestion, the SLD in flaxseeds is converted by large-bowel bacteria into two estrogen-like substances known as enterolactone and enterodiol. These are classified as phytoestrogens, or plant-based estrogens, which means they can bind to estrogen receptors on breast tissue, the endometrium of the uterus, and the cervix, moderating their overstimulation of the body's more potent estrogens. This is important because overstimulation of these tissues by endogenous estrogens (in the form of hormone replacement therapy or the birth control pill) is linked to an increased risk of breast cancer, endometrial cancer, and cancer of the cervix.

A recently published Toronto-based hospital study demonstrated that flaxseed supplementation greatly improved symptoms in women who suffered from fibrocystic breast disease. Other studies have shown that flaxseed supplementation can help normalize estrogen production and reduce the buildup of more cancer-permissive estrogens. Furthermore, it has slowed breast cell division rates, a factor in the prevention of breast cancer development. All indicators suggest that every woman over the age of 16 should capitalize on the contributions of flaxseed to the lifelong health of reproductive tissues.

Flaxseed and Prostate Health

The phytoestrogens derived from flaxseed also help preserve prostate health in various ways. First, enterolactone and enterodiol block the overproduction of estrone hormone within fat cells. With weight gain, fat cells become larger and tend to manufacture more estrone hormone, which encourages prostate cells to synthesize more dihydrotestosterone (DHT). A buildup of DHT in the prostate, in turn, stimulates rapid division of the prostate cells, leading to prostate enlargement, and accelerates the growth of any existing prostate cancer cells. By age 50, approximately 15 to 30 percent of men worldwide already have some cancer cells present within the prostate gland. Keeping DHT levels in check is vital to prevent these cancer cells from spreading throughout the prostate gland and metastasizing to other parts of the body. The ingestion of flaxseed on a daily basis provides bioactive agents that indirectly slow the rate of prostate cell replication, reducing the chances of prostate enlargement and of cancer development. These same phytoestrogens also bind to receptors on the prostate gland, blocking the influence of other hormones which can stimulate rapid prostate cell division. Herbal compounds such as saw palmetto, pygeum africanum, soy isoflavonoids and beta-sitosterol can halt the buildup of DHT as well and have improved prostate health in a number of well-designed clinical studies. Because prostate cancer is so widespread and prostate enlargement problems affect 80 percent of men who live to old age, I recommend the daily ingestion of 50 mg of ground flaxseed for every adult male.

Flaxseed and Cholesterol

Studies reveal that the same amount of flaxseed required to maintain male and female reproductive tissue health—approximately 40 to 50 mg daily—can also lower blood cholesterol by up to 10 percent in people with high cholesterol levels. More important, it lowers the bad LDL cholesterol by approximately 15 percent and concentrations of lipoprotein (a) by seven percent. Lipoprotein (a) is now recognized as a significant risk factor for heart disease, and flaxseed supplementation is the only known dietary intervention that can lower its levels into a safer range. Flaxseed contains soluble dietary fiber, which has proven cholesterol-lowering effects, plus binds to bile acids, preventing their re-absorption back into the bloodstream and subsequent conversion into cholesterol in the liver.

Flaxseed and Bowel Function

Flaxseed also contains insoluble dietary fiber, which acts as a bulking agent or roughage, encouraging more regular bowel movements. Flaxseed supplementation provides a natural and gentle laxative effect, relieving constipation and promoting the health of the large bowel. By providing both soluble and insoluble dietary fiber, flaxseed is one of the few natural nutrition products that can help to keep cholesterol levels under control and regulate bowel function at the same time.

Flaxseed and Liver and Gallbladder Support

The daily ingestion of ground flaxseed will improve the flow of bile from the liver to the gallbladder, and ultimately into the intestinal tract. This effect reduces the chances of gallstone formation and related gallbladder disease. Essentially, flaxseed supplementation induces a liver flushing effect, preventing the stagnation of bile which can harden into stones if not eliminated in a timely fashion.

Don't Confuse Flaxseed Powder with Flaxseed Oil

Consumers are often confused by the differences between flaxseed powder and flaxseed oil. Flaxseed powder (ground flaxseed) is a rich source of phytoestrogens, as well as cholesterol-cruncher and colon-cleaner fiber, and thus contributes significantly to female and male reproductive health, to the lowering of cholesterol, improved liver and gallbladder function, and regulation of the large bowel.

Flaxseed oil, on the other hand, is an abundant source of the omega-3 fat known as alpha-linolenic acid, which as we know can be converted into the highly beneficial prostaglandin series-3. Omega-3 fats, including alpha-linolenic acid, have demonstrated an ability to slow the cell replication rate of breast, prostate, and colon cells. The evidence suggests that taken together, flaxseed powder and flaxseed oil provide considerable anti-aging and disease prevention properties.

How to Use Flaxseed

You can purchase ground flaxseeds (or flaxseed powder, as it may be labelled), or you can grind whole flaxseeds in a coffee grinder to ensure its freshness. Flaxseeds or powder from organic sources are easily attainable. As suggested, two heaping tablespoons of 40 to 50 gm of ground flaxseed per day provides the health-promoting advantages described in this section. It can be mixed into a protein shake or fruit juice, sprinkled on cereal or mixed into a bowl of low-fat yogurt. It can also be added as an ingredient in low-fat muffins or take center stage in flaxbread. The important thing is that you consume at least 25 gm per day, and ideally 40 to 50 gm, by whatever delivery system works for you. The best news is that it has a nutty, flavorful taste that is palatable and very enjoyable.

Flaxseed is truly one of nature's gifts. Incorporate it into a proactive, anti-aging, disease prevention lifestyle and use it for a lifetime.

*For access to the references to Step 2 and additional education on wellness please visit the author's web site at **www.renaisante.com***

STEP 3

Commit to a Regular Exercise Program

The human body has over 600 muscles, allowing it an extraordinary range and capacity for movement. Physical exertion should be as natural to us as breathing. Yet the average North American exerts himself very little. Our activity levels have been reduced by cars, assembly lines, farm equipment, elevators, washing machines, snow blowers, and golf carts, to name only a few labour-saving and consequently movement-saving devices.

Going against our genetic programming that demands that we use our bodies in a physical way leads inevitably to disease and degeneration. The high-tech, industrialized conditions of the modern world has led to a state where for many people their bodies are simply there to carry their head from place to place. Much of a person's activity in daily life has shifted from physical activity to brain-related activity such as thinking, problem solving, goal setting, and communicating. There is no doubt that the progressive decline in physical activity over the decades has contributed to a rise in obesity, heart disease, and cancer. We have

to find twenty-first century substitutes for those physically challenging tasks we no longer need to perform. Walking, jogging,
cycling, rowing, swimming, aerobics, dancing—there are lots of
possibilities. Your body demands a certain amount of physical
activity every week; without it, you can look forward to a degenerative process that is not unlike starvation.

Even if your diet is ideal, your muscles will degenerate and
shrink without adequate exercise. They will also become more
susceptible to tears and ruptures. They will no longer adequately
support your joints, especially your hips, knees, and lower back.
You will be prone to osteoarthritis. Your bones will lose calcium
more easily, increasing your chance of developing osteoporosis.
Without adequate physical activity, you can count on progressive
deterioration of your muscle and bone structure, your cardiovascular
integrity, and other organ systems.

Exercise Prevents Age-Related Muscle and Bone Loss and Cardiovascular Decline

After the age of 40 there is a significant decline in the secretion
rates and blood levels of testosterone, dehydroepiandrosterone
(DHEA), growth hormone, and Insulin-like Growth Factor-1 (IGF-1)
in both sexes, and an additional decline in estrogen and progesterone in women entering menopause. These age-related hormonal
changes allow our muscle mass to be broken down and used to
produce energy. Decreased muscle mass contributes to a slower
metabolism and greater gains in body fat. As we age *too* these
changes *also* permit calcium to leech out of bone, increasing the
risk of osteoporosis. There is a decline in cardiovascular function.

The cells of the body become less efficient at extracting oxygen from the bloodstream, and our maximum heart rate drops. The good news is that the right combination of aerobic exercise and resistance training will prevent the loss of muscle mass and bone density and maintain cardiovascular function at a more youthful level. In fact, studies on elderly subjects have shown that aerobic exercise can improve many aspects of cardiovascular function and oxygen uptake and utilization by the cells of the body, and that a basic resistance training routine can increase muscle mass and bone density, thereby reversing the aging process. Aerobic and resistance training exercise together can allow us to attain and maintain a fit, toned, and strong body well into our twilight years.

I have been reasonably fit my whole life thanks largely to aerobics training. But at age 40 I put extra emphasis on the resistance training portion of my exercise routine—weights and strength exercises—in an effort to increase my muscle mass, tone, and definition. At this stage in life I began a regimen of one hour of moderate to heavy resistance training six days per week. I continued at least 30 minutes of aerobic exercise per day and adjusted my diet to include the additional protein I required to build more muscle. In the first two years of this program I gained up to 15 pounds of muscle and reduced my body fat by four percent. I have been able to maintain these levels for the past 10 years and have a better body now than I did in my 20's and 30's.

Like many others, I am living proof that the aging process need not leave us flabby, weak, and easily winded. Even though the hormonal changes of aging make it more challenging to achieve and maintain these results, it is absolutely within your ability to have a toned, lean body regardless of your age.

The Essentials of Aerobic Exercise

Participating in aerobic exercise may be the single most important proactive wellness strategy you can adopt. Regular aerobic exercise improves the health of your cardiovascular system, strengthens your heart muscle, burns body fat, elevates good HDL cholesterol, reduces high triglyceride levels, helps reduce high blood pressure, and regulates insulin. It is associated with a significant reduction in the risk of breast and colon cancer, and it increases the release of endorphins, which elevate your mood, reduce stress, and combat mild to moderate cases of depression.

Aerobic exercise is any activity that accelerates your heart rate to within what is known as the "aerobic training zone" for a minimum of 20 minutes (ideally, 30 to 60 minutes) and is practiced at least three times a week. This means that you should exercise at a level of intensity that has you breathing harder than normal but still able to carry on a conversation. Popular options include jogging, stationary cycling, rowing, long-distance swimming, cross-country skiing, working out on elliptical machines, Stair Masters, Stair Climbers, and aerobic fitness or dance classes. All of these forms of exercise offer the health benefits I've described.

Achieving your aerobic training heart-rate zone is the key. Essentially, this zone is between 60 and 85 percent of your maximum attainable heart rate. This is the rate at which your heart would beat if you were to exercise all-out, to the point of complete exhaustion. Fortunately, you don't have to reach this point. You can determine your aerobic zone by making a few simple calculations, beginning with your maximum attainable heart rate.

- Maximum attainable heart rate = 220 minus your age
- Low end of aerobic heart-rate zone = maximum attainable heart rate x 0.6
- High end of aerobic heart-rate zone = maximum attainable heart rate x 0.85

If you are 40 years old, your maximum attainable heart rate is approximately 180 beats per minute (220 - 40). Your aerobic heart-rate zone ranges from 108 beats per minute (180 x 0.6) to 153 beats per minute (180 x 0.85). You will get the most aerobic exercise by keeping your heart rate at between 108 and 153 beats per minute for 20 to 45 minutes, at least three times a week.

Exercising at 60 percent of your maximum attainable rate is so comfortable that you can maintain a conversation without becoming winded. If you are just starting with aerobic exercise, you should aim for about 65 percent of your maximum attainable rate. If you are already in good shape, aim for at least 75 percent. You can push yourself harder by doing short sprint intervals during your aerobic workout. I'll explain interval training later in this section.

You will be amazed at how quickly your body responds to a regular aerobics program. I have seen many patients who were seriously overweight or out of shape achieve remarkable results in short periods of time. I have seen first-time joggers who took ten or eleven minutes to complete a mile improve their times to eight, seven, or even an elite-level six minutes a mile. These gains are due to an increase in the muscles' oxygen consumption and in the number of sites within the muscle that can generate energy. With more available energy, the muscles can do more work, enabling you to run faster or row harder or cycle uphill at the same heart rate at which you previously performed to a lesser degree.

Maximal heart rates and training sensitive zones for use in aerobic training programs for people of different ages

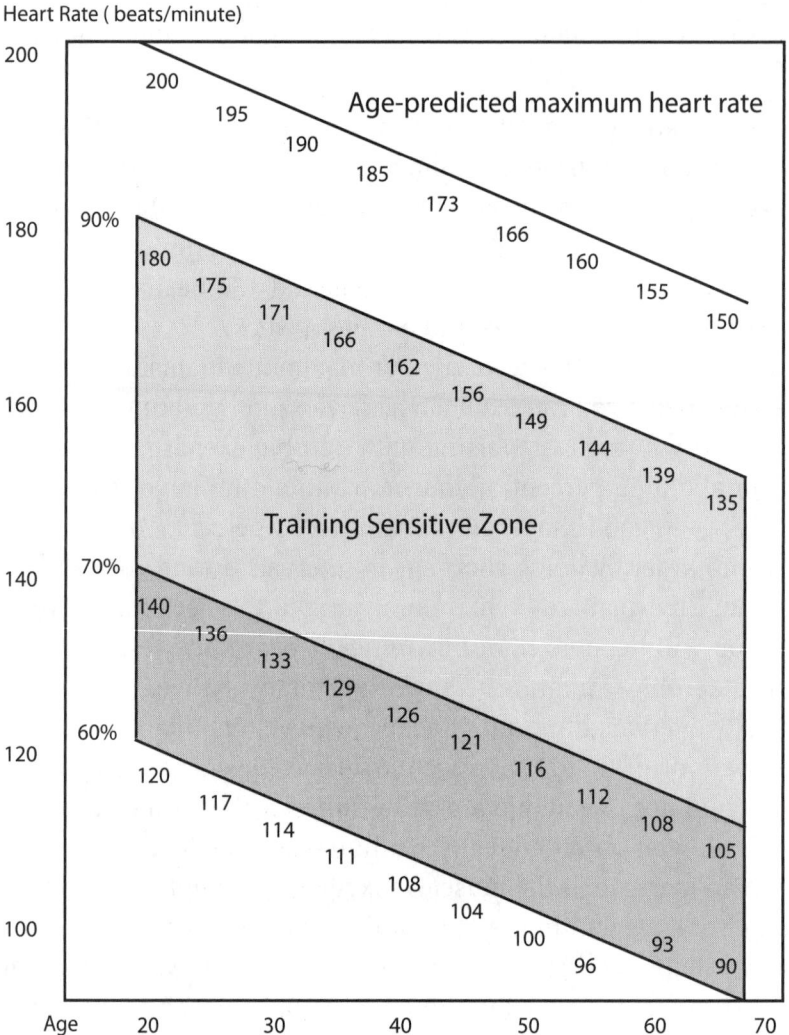

Heart Rate (beats/minute)

The zone between 60 and 70 percent of your maximum heart rate is sufficient to derive aerobic benefits and at the same time is not so demanding as to produce significant discomfort.

Your overall aerobic exercise performance will gradually improve as a result of regular participation. You don't have to overexert yourself: your speed, endurance, and strength will increase as a natural response to the aerobic exercise itself.

Aerobic exercise improves the capacity of your body tissues to extract oxygen from red blood cells, transport it to the inside of the cells, and use it for energy production. Although your red blood cells are always saturated with more oxygen than your body requires at any given moment, the ability of the tissues to pick up this oxygen can vary greatly from one person to the next. An aerobically fit individual extracts oxygen from the bloodstream roughly 25 percent more efficiently than someone who is unfit. Light activity alone will not significantly improve the utilization of oxygen in your body. You must maintain an increased heart rate for at least 20 minutes three times a week to make these positive changes. In just six to eight weeks, the average person can increase his or her oxygen consumption by 10 to 15 percent through aerobic exercise.

The benefits of improved oxygen utilization are considerable: you will have more energy; your tissues will become more efficient at using the oxygen available, so your heart will be under less stress; your heart will become stronger and able to pump more blood with every beat. Thus, it can beat more slowly and still provide adequate blood to your body. On average, an aerobically fit person actually has a slower resting heart rate (48 to 66 beats per minute) than an aerobically unfit person (72 to 99 beats per minute).

A slower resting heart beat is a tremendous advantage in itself. Between beats, your heart can deliver blood to its own coronary vessels and supply itself with more oxygen. To appreciate the importance of these aerobic adaptations, keep in mind that a heart attack occurs when your heart muscle cannot get the oxygen it needs. The better your heart is equipped to deliver oxygen to its own muscles, the better off you are. But that's not all. Studies show that aerobically fit exercisers have higher levels of HDL cholesterol, the "good" cholesterol that helps prevent the arteries from narrowing and may even reverse the narrowing process.

Furthermore, aerobic exercise lowers psychological stress by balancing and regulating hormones that promote high blood pressure. In periods of stress, the amount of adrenaline hormone in your system increases. During aerobic exercise, your body releases adrenaline slowly and regularly; after exercising, your level of adrenaline returns to the ideal baseline.

Many highly stressed people have discovered that aerobic exercise helps them unwind. It's a great way to clear the cobwebs from your head and put the anxieties of the day into perspective. In fact, aerobic exercise can take you into an altered state of consciousness that triggers positive thoughts. It is well documented that exercise helps prevent recurring depression and at the same time induces runner's high, the heightened mood that usually kicks in after 20 to 30 minutes of an aerobic workout session. Research indicates that this state is created by the release of pleasure-giving brain chemicals know as endorphins.

Finally, exercise affects your appetite and food choices. Most people find it easier to make wise food choices after an exercise routine. The appetite center seems to prefer healthier, lighter foods. And losing a few extra pounds through aerobic exercise can also help lower your blood pressure and reduce your risk of cardiovascular disease.

You can be trim and slender but still unfit from an aerobic point of view. Conversely, you can be in great aerobic shape even if you are overweight. No matter how much you weigh, you can achieve great benefits to your heart, cardiovascular system, and muscle tissues from aerobic exercise. Being aerobically fit actually helps minimize some of the risks of being overweight, so don't wait to lose weight before you begin an aerobic exercise program.

Spot-reducing exercises such as sit-ups and leg lifts will tone the muscles under the fat, but they will not eliminate fat itself. Only aerobic exercise can stimulate the release of fat from your fat cells. Here's how it works. Let's say you get on a stationary bicycle and begin peddling. As your heart beat speeds up, your nervous system releases adrenaline. Adrenaline triggers the breakdown of fat in fat cells everywhere in your body, not in the muscles you are exercising. Individual fat molecules escape from your fat cells and enter the bloodstream, where they circulate through your body. The exercising muscles, including the heart and respiratory muscles, pick up the circulating fat molecules and burn them to generate energy. The longer you peddle the more fat is released and burned.

When you stop exercising your tissues will very quickly stop releasing fat molecules into your bloodstream. However, your muscles will continue to pick up and burn the fat already there. Several factors affect how long you burn fat after exercise. Most significantly, the longer the exercise session, the more fat will be released from your fat cells and therefore the more fat is burned after exercise. Ideally, you should build up to sessions of between 30 and 60 minutes' duration. A 30 to 60 minute session also markedly depletes the carbohydrate stores in your muscles and liver. Your body will be so busy rebuilding these stores that most of your tissue cells will continue to burn fat as their primary fuel for many hours after the workout is over.

The Essentials of Resistance Training

With a routine of aerobic exercise established, I recommend that you add resistance training—strength and weight training—to your fitness program. Resistance training will give you muscle tone and definition, improve body shaping and strength, and raise your metabolic rate, enabling your body to burn more fat calories while you are at rest. Resistance training also helps you gain bone mass, which prevents osteoporosis. And like aerobic exercise, resistance training greatly depletes the carbohydrate stores in the muscles exercised. When the exercise session is over for the day, your tissue cells will primarily burn fat, as your body shunts the carbohydrate calories you consume to your muscles so they can reload their carbohydrate fuel tank in preparation for your next work out. Finally, resistance training, performed properly, improves your posture and helps prevent sprains, strains, and injuries to your muscle and joint systems.

Resistance training is best performed with free weights or resistance training machines. If you are unfamiliar with this equipment or the names of the exercises, seek some basic instruction from a fitness professional or personal trainer at a gym. These strength training exercises are easy to learn and the equipment is safe for almost everyone.

If you are just beginning an aerobic exercise program and have been unfit for some time, you may not be ready to embrace resistance training right away. However, when you become more experienced and fit, I suggest you adopt one of the programs described later in this chapter or ask a fitness instructor at a local health club to design a routine that is customized for your needs.

In recent years weight training or resistance training has become increasingly popular with athletes in every sport and fitness-conscious individuals of all ages. Gone are the days when the weight room was the exclusive domain of Olympic weight lifters, body builders, and muscle heads. Today, many recreational athletes and fitness enthusiasts recognize the performance-enhancing, body-shaping and even medicinal value of weight training.

Successful resistance training begins with identifying your goal. If you want a body builder's physique, then follow a program that maximizes muscle growth and density. If you're trying to improve the power of your tennis stroke, your slap shot, your bat speed in baseball, your golf swing, your skating power or your speed and acceleration for soccer or sprinting, then using a body builder's weight training routine may actually slow you down and worsen your performance. You might get bigger, but you'll probably be slower. The explanation lies in an understanding of muscle mechanics.

One of the body's fundamental adaptations to weight training is an increase in muscle fiber size, a condition known as hypertrophy. The number of muscle fibers in the muscle doesn't increase. Rather, the muscle fibers simply lay down more protein myofilaments (actin and myosin protein) in their outer layers. A muscle like your biceps, for instance, is made up of thousands of individual muscle fibers, each about the diameter of a human hair. As you train these muscles through resistance training, they respond by enlarging, laying down an increased number of myofilaments inside each trained muscle fiber, thus increasing their cross-sectional area and their density. As the cross-sectional area of the muscle increases, its maximum force or strength increases, and the muscle begins to look more toned, better defined. These adaptations hold true for both men and women.

However, muscle fiber hypertrophy does not occur uniformly among all the fibers in the exercised muscle. In every muscle, there are Slow Twitch (Type I) and Fast Twitch (Type II) muscle fibers. Slow Twitch fibers are aerobic in nature, designed for high oxygen consumption, and are recruited primarily for long distance or endurance-based activities. Fast Twitch fibers are needed for explosive bursts of energy (golf swings, tennis strokes, sprinting, etc.). Some people are genetically endowed with a greater number of Fast Twitch fibers than others and have a natural ability to run fast or hit a golf ball a country mile with little or no formal training. The resistance training programs that I will outline produce hypertrophy primarily in Fast Twitch fibers, rather than in Slow Twitch fibers.

Body builders focus on both Type I and Type II muscle fiber hypertrophy. As a rule, Type I muscle fibers resist increasing in size. This is why long distance runners do not look muscular, even though their Type I muscle fibers are extremely fit and well trained. Body builders have discovered that they can force Type I muscle fiber to grow by including high-volume, low-resistance training in their workout programs. This enables them to gain the bulky muscles that we associate with body builders.

For the rest of us, a resistance training program will be based on a series of weight-bearing exercises performed with six or seven pieces of weight training equipment. Each exercise is performed with a specific weight and for a specific number of sets and repetitions within a set. To improve muscle definition, body sculpting, strength and power, choose a weight that you can lift eight to 10 times. Then perform three to five sets of eight to 10 repetitions each with this weight. It should be heavy enough that you are unable to do more than 10 repetitions in a set. Rest for a minute or two between sets. While performing the exercise, contract the muscle quickly when working against the resistance, then lower the weight in a slow, controlled manner. Rapid contraction against the weight helps improve muscle power, increases your speed and acceleration, and recruits a greater number of total muscle fibers into the effort. Lowering slowly will reduce the strain on joint structures.

Once you can lift the weight 10 times in each of the four or five sets at that exercise station, make the weight heavier on your next visit to the gym. Continue to increase the weight as your muscles become stronger, always working towards 10 repetitions in each set. This is known as the overload principle of resistance training, a technique that enables your muscle strength gains, body sculpting, and definition to continue improving over time.

To maximize your weight training results, follow these tips:

- Perform at least two or three different exercises for each body part. For the chest, as an example, use the bench press, incline press, and flies;

- Perform three to five sets at each exercise station.

- Work each body part at least twice a week allowing 48 to 72 hours for recovery between sessions;

- To achieve greater strength gains, use heavier weights that permit you to perform only four to seven repetitions per set, before reaching muscular failure;

- For power training to enhance sports performance, body sculpting and general anti-aging purposes, use moderate weights and eight to 10 repetitions per set to muscular failure;

- Remember that to gain muscle mass you must ingest at least 0.5 grams of protein for every pound you weigh (or about 1.2 grams of protein for every kilogram you weigh). Some athletes ingest up to 2.2 grams of protein per kg. As an example, if you weigh 80 kilograms, you should consider ingesting 100 to 150 grams of protein each day to build your muscles depending on the intensity, duration, and frequency of your workouts.

For Those Who Hate to Exercise

Does the very thought of aerobic exercise exhaust you? Do you regard resistance training as not only painful but painfully boring? I have met many individuals who feel this way. Despite the phenomenal growth of the wellness movement in the past twenty-five years, many people are still reluctant to undertake even a moderate exercise regimen.

Perhaps you are among them, although you acknowledge the health risks of a couch potato lifestyle. My advice is start small: you can attain some of the benefits of regular exercise through a program of relatively light activity, such as walking. Several studies have shown that burning 2000 calories per week with easy physical activity increases longevity. This expenditure, achieved by walking alone, has been shown by researchers to lower the risk of coronary heart disease by as much as 39 percent, even in overweight smokers with high blood pressure. We're not talking about sweat and exertion here: most people can burn 2000 calories during a walk of 45 to 60 minutes (three to four miles, or five to 6.5 km) four to six times a week.

Other research has demonstrated that light regular physical activity is linked to the prevention of colon cancer and decreases in breast cancer, the latter thanks to its influence on estrogen levels. During a woman's teenage years, excess body fat can establish a pattern of estrogen secretion that may hasten the onset of cancers in the reproductive tissues later in life. When fat cells increase in size because of overeating and lack of exercise, they can become over-stimulated and increase the production of potentially harmful forms of estrogen. Dr. Rose Frisch, a researcher at the Harvard School of Public Health, Center for Population Studies, studied the prevalence (lifetime occurrence) rates of reproductive organ cancers in women based upon data collected from 5,398 living alumnae, 2,622 of whom were former college athletes and 2,776 nonathletes. Participants (former alumnae) were mailed a detailed questionnaire dealing with their health history from 1981–82 up until 1996–97—a 15-year follow up period. She found that women who have exercised over their lifetimes have a dramatically lower rate of reproductive organ cancers than women with histories of little exercise.

Any way you look at it, the message is clear. Physical activity need not be excessively demanding for it to be of some value in the prevention of heart disease and cancer. However, more formalized aerobic exercise provides greater total benefits—anti-aging, disease prevention, fitness, and body shaping and toning. The chances are that once you start, you'll want those too.

Choosing the Right Program

I will offer you five different exercise programs to choose from, according to your present fitness level, health status, health history, wellness and anti-aging goals, and time constraints:

1. The Power Walk Program—a light activity program for people who hate to exercise;

2. The Basic Aerobic Program—an aerobic program to ensure that you derive all the benefits available from aerobic exercise;

3. The Aerobic Plus Basic 6 Resistance Training Program—the basic aerobic program plus a starter program of resistance training, which provides the six most important resistance exercises for the upper and lower body;

4. Aerobic Plus Intermediate Resistance Training Program—the basic aerobic program plus an intermediate program of resistance training;

5. Aerobic Plus Advanced Split Routine Resistance Training Program—the basic aerobic program with a more advanced program of resistance training for even better results in body shaping, muscle tone, definition, and strength.

1—The Power Walk Program

By burning as few as 2000 calories per week, you can improve your wellbeing whether you want to lose weight or not. How can you burn off 2000 calories? Here is a helpful formula: by walking one kilometre, you burn as many calories as you weigh in kilograms. If you weigh 70 kg, you will burn roughly 70 calories by walking a kilometre. Let's say you walk five kilometres (three miles) a day, six times a week: 70 calories x 5 km x 6 times per week = 2100 calories. That is enough physical activity to significantly decrease your risks of heart disease and certain cancers.

If you wish, you can jog some of those kilometers instead of walking them. The main difference between walking and jogging is your time to the finish line. Jogging will provide some additional aerobic benefits, but walking should not be underrated as a method of exercise. You'll burn the same number of calories as you do jogging and you can do it almost anywhere with no need for fancy equipment. Keep up a brisk steady pace—you're not out for a stroll, you're out for a power walk.

Wear a proper pair of shoes, preferably jogging shoes with good support. Choose different routes to keep your walks interesting. Listen to your favorite music to help maintain your pace or to an audiobook to make double use of your time. You can plan a party, compose a letter, or rehearse a presentation while you walk. To burn even more calories, carry one-pound hand weights or wrist weights. By swinging your arms energetically as you walk, you will further increase your heart rate, making the power walk more of an aerobic workout. Jazz dancing and ballroom dancing are good supplements to the power walk program. One hour of dancing is roughly equivalent to a three-mile walk.

Eventually, you will probably find the power walk is not enough of a challenge. This means you're getting into shape. Try alternating walking and jogging. Jog until you feel tired, then walk until you recover. Don't be surprised when one day you find yourself able to jog the entire distance.

2—The Basic Aerobic Program

Any activity that keeps your heart beating within your aerobic training heart-rate zone is good aerobic exercise, whether it's jogging, cycling, rowing, or just running up and down the stairs. Fitness classes can be an effective form of aerobic exercise as well, as long as they maintain your heart rate within the aerobic heart-rate zone for more than 20 minutes. Classes such as cardio-pump and body sculpting can also improve muscle-toning, strength and flexibility and serve as great overall conditioners. Nonetheless, I suggest that you complement these classes with some additional aerobic and strength training work on your own.

If you have not exercised for a long time, consult your doctor before embarking on an ambitious aerobic program. Begin with 20-minute exercise sessions and gradually work up to 45 to 60 minutes. A 45 to 60 minute session maximizes the amount of fat you will continue to burn after exercising.

To derive the major aerobic benefits of jogging, you should cover at least 15 miles (24 km) per week. If you jog more than 25 miles (40 km) per week, however, you may put yourself at risk for the development of shin splints, ankle problems, or knee problems. Measure other forms of aerobic exercise, such as swimming or working out on stationary bikes, rowing machines, cross-country machines, treadmills, mini-trampolines, and stair climbers, by the length of time you spend on them, not by the "distance" you cover. What matters is the length of time that your heart rate stays within your aerobic training heart-rate zone. If you are training three days a week, these days should not be consecutive. You need to train every second day to sustain the training effect. Don't push yourself to exhaustion. Make exercise something you enjoy.

Add Interval Training to Your Aerobic Workout to Enhance Power and Fat Burning

Once you become more aerobically fit, you can add interval training to your aerobic work out if it serves your goals. Interval training enables you to become better conditioned for many endurance and stop-and-go sports and to burn more fat and calories during and after your aerobic workout session. Let's take a look at interval training and whether it suits your needs.

The key to success in many sports is the ability to repeatedly attain high speed and sustain it for extended periods of time. This is especially true of sports played over large surfaces—hockey rinks, basketball courts, football or soccer fields, singles tennis courts, or middle distance track and field events. We've all seen a ball carrier in football slow down within 10 or 15 yards of the goal posts after a 70 or 80 yard breakaway run. He has dodged and sprinted his way through the opposition, but then begins to fatigue. A better-conditioned defending player catches up and makes the tackle, ending his hopes of a touchdown.

With some minor adjustments to your aerobic training routine you can stimulate your muscles to improve your speed endurance. Even if you're not the fastest athlete on the field, being able to sustain your maximum speed for the necessary length of time will often give you an edge over the naturally faster athlete who lacks speed endurance capacity.

On the two or three days a week that you do your aerobic workout incorporate a few minutes of interval training. Instead of jogging or cycling or using a Stair Master at a constant pace within your aerobic heart rate zone, set aside 10 to 15 minutes of your usual training period to include short interval sprints, followed by a less demanding recovery interval. The sprint phase of high intensity work should closely match the peak demands of your sport and the recovery phase should likewise mimic the recovery interval of your sport. Here are a few approximate sprint to recovery intervals for various sports:

- Football: 20 to 30 seconds sprint phase followed by 60 seconds of recovery within your low to moderate aerobic range.

- Basketball: 20 to 30 seconds sprint followed by 60 seconds of recovery within your low to moderate aerobic range.

- Baseball: 40 seconds sprint followed by 90 seconds of recovery within your low to moderate aerobic range.

- Soccer: 30 seconds sprint followed by 60 seconds of recovery within your low to moderate aerobic range.

- Hockey and ringette: 30 seconds sprint followed by 60 to 90 seconds of recovery within your low to moderate aerobic range.

- Lacrosse: 30 seconds sprint followed by 60 seconds of recovery within your low to moderate aerobic range.

Keep in mind that the sprint interval requires all-out or near all-out effort. During the recovery interval, keep moving, but reduce your speed or the resistance of the machine so you can prepare for the next sprint interval. When beginning to train this way, perform only six to eight sprints during your aerobic session. As you become better conditioned you can increase the number of sprint intervals to eight to 15 per session.

Interval training takes your aerobic fitness capacity to a whole new level, which translates into better performance and a more fit-looking, fat-burning body.

3 — The Aerobic Plus Basic 6 Resistance Training Program

This program comprises your usual aerobic exercise program and a resistance training program that works all of the major muscle groups in the body with only six exercises, three for the upper body and three for the lower. It is a great program if you have not done resistance training before.

Exercise	Sets	Repetitions		
		First set	Second set	Third set
Bench or Chest Press	3	8-10	8	8
Lat Pull Downs	3	8-10	8	8
Overhead Press	3	8-10	8	8
Hip Extension (or Squats)	3	8-10	8	8
Knee Extension	3	8-10	8	8
Hamstring Curl	3	8-10	8	8

Your goal is to perform this strength training program three or four times per week, which will accelerate your strength gains, your muscle tone, and your body shaping. Allow at least 48 hours between training sessions. It's during the recovery days that your muscles rebuild themselves with a greater number of fibers.

Strength training is now an integral part of life for most fitness and wellness-conscious individuals. If you are serious about achieving a healthy, fit, toned body, then I encourage you to adopt this beginner-level strengthening program. You will be amazed at how quickly your strength, performance, and muscle tone improve.

4—The Aerobic Plus Intermediate Resistance Training Program

This program comprises your usual aerobic training program plus three or four sessions a week of a nine-exercise resistance training regimen.

Exercise	Sets	Repetitions		
		First set	Second set	Third set
Bench Press	3	8-10	8-10	8-10
Incline Press	3	8-10	8-10	8-10
Lateral Pull Downs	3	8-10	8-10	8-10
Seated Rowing	3	8-10	8-10	8-10
Squats	3	8-10	8-10	8-10
Knee Extension	3	8-10	8-10	8-10
Hamstring Curl	3	8-10	8-10	8-10
Bicep Curl	3	8-10	8-10	8-10
Tricep Extension	3	8-10	8-10	8-10

5—The Aerobic Plus Advanced Split Routine Resistance Training Program

This program combines your usual aerobic exercise routine with a more advanced resistance training program.

Follow the Day 1 routine, then Day 2. On the third day, take a day off from weight training to allow full recovery. On the fourth day, return to the Day 1 routine. This gives you a rest every third day from your weight training program.

Day 1 - Chest, Back and Biceps

Exercise	Sets	Repetitions		
		First set	Second set	Third set
Bench Press	3	6-8	6-8	6-8
Incline Press	3	6-8	6-8	6-8
Flies	3	6-8	6-8	6-8
Lateral Pul Downs	3	6-8	6-8	6-8
Seated Rowing	3	6-8	6-8	6-8
Bicep Curls	3	6-8	6-8	6-8

Day 2 - Legs, Shoulders and Triceps

Exercise	Sets	Repetitions		
		First set	Second set	Third set
Squats	3	6-8	6-8	6-8
Knee Extension	3	6-8	6-8	6-8
Hamstring Curl	3	6-8	6-8	6-8
Military Press	3	6-8	6-8	6-8
Lateral Raises	3	6-8	6-8	6-8
Upright Rowing	3	6-8	6-8	6-8
Tricep Extensions	3	6-8	6-8	6-8

There are many variations of this training method and you may wish to consult a personal trainer for more individualized or sports-specific programs.

Other Resistance Training Exercises That Work

In my experience there are alternative programs to traditional weight training that also enhance muscle strength, definition, tone and body shape. Specific exercises using the Thera-Ball can be very useful and are easily performed in your own home. Have a trainer devise a personalized routine for you using this piece of equipment. Other effective programs to investigate include:

- Yoga – especially Ashtanga, Bikram, and power yoga
- Body sculpting and body-pump fitness classes
- Martial arts training
- Pilates
- Boxercise

If you are involved in these alternate forms of resistance training, I recommend supplementing them with Program 3: The Basic 6 Resistance Training Program, at least twice per week.

Long-Term Compliance

Still see exercise as an unpleasant and uncomfortable chore? If so, you need to learn how to make it fun. Exercising should give you the same feeling of revitalization as dancing. I recommended taped music for power walking, but it's appropriate to any form of aerobic exercise. Listening to favourite songs will make continuous movement feel natural and an upbeat tempo can spur you to greater heights.

At the outset of an exercise program, you will probably have to take firm charge of your body. Deprived of regular physical activity, it will be weak, tired, and addicted to the foods and behaviors that have kept you out of shape. Listening to your body at this point won't do you any good. It will dictate terms that favour the status quo. As Newton so aptly stated, "A body at rest stays at rest." You must, therefore, commit to a fitness goal and know how you can accomplish it, beginning with fitting exercise into your schedule. What works best for you? A morning walk? An evening jog? Perhaps a workout at lunchtime? Make your exercise times convenient, so that you will be more inclined to stick to them.

If your body remains reluctant, then it's up to your mind to force it into action. Exercise even when you don't feel like it. In a matter of minutes both your body and mind will feel better. I guarantee it. Improved psychological wellbeing is one of the major benefits of exercise. Take advantage of the runner's high, that pleasurable sensation that arises during your aerobic workout. View your exercise time as wellness time—time to clear your head, move your body, and recharge your battery. Physical activity can literally change your mood. Learn to anticipate the positive feelings of wellbeing that come from exercising. Don't let glum days, hectic days, or boring days get you down. Exercise is an excellent way to leave those self-destructive emotions behind and get on with the happy, positive life you deserve.

Remember it's not about pushing yourself to exhaustion. A patient who came to me overweight and out of shape now runs marathons several times a year. When he jogs, he concentrates on the idea of conserving his energy. He never pushes himself to the point of pain or exhaustion because he knows that he will have a negative reaction, physically and psychologically. "I want to wake up tomorrow and look forward to my exercise session. I don't want to dread it," he says. If you push yourself too hard, it makes sense that you would be tired and resentful about exercising the next time. And your psychological outlook and day-to-day energy have everything to do with staying on track.

How do you know you won't enjoy a regular exercise program if you don't try it? Give yourself a chance to experience the physical and mental benefits. I predict that exercise will become a positive and permanent feature in your life and that you will come to rely on it as an essential source of rejuvenation.

Starting Right Now...

1. Decide to stick with an exercise program for at least eight consecutive weeks.

2. Choose the exercise program that is right for you: Program 1, 2, 3, 4, or 5.

3. Visit your doctor before starting. Find out whether she or he recommends a stress test, electrocardiogram, or other exam before you begin an exercise regimen.

*For access to the references to Step 3 and additional education on wellness please visit the author's web site at **www.renaisante.com***

STEP 4

Follow the Two Staple Nutrition System

By now you are aware of the essential ingredients of a health-promoting diet, the benefits of lifelong supplementation, and the rewards of a regular exercise plan that suits your particular circumstances. Step 4 is to incorporate the wellness principles you have learned into a simple yet effective system of eating that will deliver the healthy body nature intended you to have. My Two Staple Nutrition System is a practical, easy-to-follow formula that puts your nutritional knowledge into action. Its flexible structure allows you to choose the foods and recipes that best suit your taste preferences and lifestyle, so that you won't feel deprived or discouraged. By designing a system that is both simple and realistic, I was able to reach my own goals and have helped many of my clients attain lean, fit, age-resistant bodies while still enjoying their daily lives. Let's get started.

The Two Staple Nutrition System

There are only two food staples to focus on under this system: protein foods and carbohydrate foods.

Protein foods, as you know, provide the building blocks of the body's structure: its muscles, bone, skin, hair, and nails. They are vital to the optimal performance of the immune system and the manufacture of specialized body proteins. On this program you will consume a low-fat protein selection at every meal, and one low-fat dairy protein selection and one low-fat flesh protein selection each at lunch and dinner. These three servings will provide most of the protein you need every day, along with the bulk of your calcium, vitamin D, iron, and vitamin B12 requirements.

The second staple is carbohydrate foods, which are converted into the glucose that powers every cell in the body. By ingesting carbohydrates in moderation and adhering to an exercise program, you will prevent the conversion of carbohydrates into fat. As described in Step 2, the right amount of carbohydrate foods can actually encourage weight loss, and Category 1, 2, and 3 carbohydrates are high in dietary fiber and other protective nutrients that help defend against cancer, heart disease, macular degeneration, cataracts, and other diseases.

Except for your intake of oils used in food preparation and salad dressings, there's no need for strict regulation of the portion sizes on this program. Eat the amount of food that your body tells you it needs, and consume the amount of protein you require based on the information presented in Step 1. At the same time, it is critically important that you don't overeat. Only you know how fast or slow your metabolism functions and how much food you can eat without gaining weight. For those who want to lose weight, I have created an intensive weight loss version of the Two Staple Nutrition System that explains the exact portion sizes for every meal. For all others your job is to pay attention to your body's responses so that you can determine the amount of food, especially carbohydrate foods, that makes you feel good and stay lean.

PROTEIN FOOD

Flesh Protein:
- chicken breast (skin removed),
- turkey breast (skin removed),
- Cornish game hens,
- fish and seafood,
- soy products such as tofu and veggie burgers.

Dairy Protein:
- low-fat cheese (less than 4% M.F.),
- plain yogurt (less than 2% M. F.),
- milk (less than 2% M. F.),
- egg whites,
- protein shake (whey-, egg white-, or soy-based).

Carbohydrate Foods:
- Category 1 carbohydrates—should comprise 40 to 45 percent of your carbohydrate intake each day.
- Category 2 carbohydrates—should comprise 20 to 25 percent of your carbohydrate intake each day.
- Category 3 and 4 carbohydrates—should comprise 20 to 25 percent of your carbohydrate intake each day, with most coming from Category 3.
- Category 5 carbohydrates—should comprise no more than 15 percent of your carbohydrate intake each day.

The Two Staple Nutrition System Meal Plan

With this plan, you eat three meals a day. At each meal you choose a protein food and surround it with two or three carbohydrate foods. For breakfast your protein staple comes from a low-fat dairy selection. If you are lactose intolerant, I suggest a lactose-free, low-fat dairy alternative; egg whites or try the protein shake option.

For lunch and dinner choose a protein food from the low-fat flesh protein selections, and surround them with two or three carbohydrate foods. You may also eat between-meal snacks judiciously from the list of solution-substitutions.

THREE MEALS PER DAY	
1. Breakfast	one low-fat dairy selection (Dairy Protein Meal): plus two carbohydrate selections.
2. Lunch	one low-fat flesh protein (Flesh Protein Meal): selection plus two to three carbohydrate selections.
3. Dinner	one low-fat flesh protein (Flesh Protein Meal):selection plus two to three carbohydrate selections.

For Vegetarians and Soy Lovers

Vegetarians can substitute different soy products for the flesh protein meal, as can non-vegetarians who are trying to include more soy in their diets, something I encourage. Most soybean products are moderately high in protein, but you should eat them with beans, peas, or grain products such as rice, bread, or pasta, for additional protein. Tofu, miso, tempeh, and texturized vegetable proteins are all reasonable sources. Vegetarians should be sure to take the multiple vitamin and mineral formula outlined in Step 2.

Soy milk can substitute for a low-fat dairy selection in the morning, but keep in mind that even fortified soy milk does not contain the amount of calcium found in cow's milk and is not usually fortified with vitamin D. A high-potency multivitamin and mineral that contains 500 mg of elemental calcium and 400 IU of vitamin D is mandatory for individuals using these soy substitutes. In many cases further supplementation with a calcium and magnesium supplement may be warranted to acquire the 1000 to 1500 mg of calcium required, depending on gender and stage of life.

Three Other Components to Track Daily

As well as consuming one dairy-protein meal and two flesh protein meals every day, you must monitor your intake of three other elements: oil, water, and fiber.

Oils

Incorporate one to two teaspoons of monounsaturated oil to your diet daily for the health-promoting benefits provided by these fats and to acquire the bit of linoleic acid an essential fat the body needs—they contain. Mix olive oil with vinegar to make salad dressings or use it to sauté vegetables or brown poultry.

The rest of the fat in your diet will come from the small amounts that are present in the low-fat dairy and flesh protein selections, as well as in some of the solution-substitution snacks and treats I will describe shortly.

Water

Try to drink at least six to eight glasses of fluids every day. If possible, drink distilled water or water that has undergone a process of reverse osmosis and deionization. Some of your fluid intake can be soda water, mineral water, or water from a deep spring.

Fiber

As we saw in Step 1, there are two equally essential kinds of fiber: cholesterol crunchers and colon cleaners. Cholesterol crunchers help keep blood cholesterol levels low, and colon cleaners dilute the effects of cancer-causing agents that may be present in the colon and rectum.

How can you be sure you are eating enough fiber? The Fiber Scoreboard (Appendix 1) will help answer that question. Drawing on the findings of two prominent researchers, Dr. D.A. Southgate and Dr. J. W. Anderson, I have reviewed the fiber content of the most common foods containing cholesterol crunchers or colon cleaners. Each has been given a point value, or score. A medium apple, for example, scores one fiber point, while half a cup of kidney beans scores three. Every point is the equivalent of three grams of fiber.

I recommend the consumption of eight to 15 fiber points every day. This amount is based on the guidelines set out by the Canadian and American cancer societies, the American Heart Society, and the Heart and Stroke Foundation. Focus most of your carbohydrate intake on Category 1, 2, and 3 carbohydrate choices, and ingest two tablespoons of flaxseed powder a day, as described in Step 2. Eating a high-fiber breakfast cereal, low-fat popcorn, beans and peas, broccoli, and apples are great ways to attain a higher fiber score every day. Additional fiber can be acquired from pysillium husk fiber supplementation.

Those eight to 15 fiber points constitute a daily prescription for keeping cholesterol levels down, glucose and insulin levels regulated, and the intestinal tract functioning properly. Keep the Fiber Scoreboard handy and consult it often. You will soon learn which are the high-fiber foods. Note your total daily fiber points to see how you're doing.

Snack, Treats, and How to Cheat

The reality is that however well-intentioned, virtually everyone will occasionally indulge in snack foods or desserts. From my experience with hundreds of patients over the years, I can tell you that most people are willing to give up high-fat animal products and switch to chicken, turkey, fish, and low-fat dairy items. But when it comes to snacks, treats, and desserts, many people lose control all too easily and undermine their whole wellness program. This is a major stumbling block to overcome, but there is a strategy to beat these cravings—one that has worked successfully for my patients and myself.

When it comes to treats and food in general, there are two types of people in this world. There are those who experience an overwhelming craving for a snack of some kind when they feel anxious, bored, depressed, or upset, or just arrive at a place in the day where they feel the need of a break before carrying on with the tasks at hand. Understand that this craving has nothing to do with hunger; it is emotionally driven. There are others who cannot eat a thing if they are anxious, depressed, upset, etc. About 80 percent of us fall into the former category. For us, eating a snack is emotionally soothing, which drives us to eat when confronted by an emotional trigger of any kind. On a subconscious level we associate the pleasure of eating with an easing of our anxiety, or a relief from tedium—or we just need the gratification of a tasty treat working over our taste buds. In our fast-paced world, most of us experience some chronic stress, and the impulse to comfort or reward ourselves at certain points in the day is a common behavior.

If this is your nature too, then understand that it will always be so. No diet plan or miracle cure is going to change this aspect of your relationship with food. It's more important to know what you can do in these moments of temptation to prevent yourself from sabotaging your wellness and weight-loss goals. The best thing you can do, of course, is realize that you are not really hungry and so not eat anything. Maybe a cup of green tea will get you through the moment. The next best thing is to eat an apple or a low-calorie/high-fiber fruit or veggie snack, but this may not work all the time either. At the very least, though, you can confront temptation with alternatives to snacks that are loaded with fat— with what I call solution-substitutions.

Solution-substitution snack foods are primarily carbohydrate-based and contain little total fat and saturated fat. Solution-substitutions are the choices to make at moments of temptation when you just can't resist. I admit that they don't taste as good as their high-fat counterparts, but it's worth making the adjustment to these kinds of comfort foods to win the anti-aging and wellness game. My patients have found it easier to remember these solution-substitution snacks and treats by categorizing them as Ooey-Gooey, Chippy-Dippy, Frozen Desserts, and Bars. Here are the in-the-moment, solution-substitution choices available to you:

SOLUTION-SUBSTITUTIONS

High-Risk Foods	Substitutions
1. Ooey-Gooey cheese cake, chocolate cake, apple pastries, doughnuts	angel food cake, muffins, pie filling (cut away the crust), fresh fruit, bagels, cinnamon raisin bread, low-fat cookies such as Fig Newtons, ginger snaps, or graham crackers
2. Chippy-Dippy potato chips, nacho chips, cheese twists, peanuts	melba toast, low-fat biscuits with salsa, rice crackers, low-fat popcorn (less than 1.5 grams fat/3cups), pretzels, roasted chestnuts
3. Frozen Desserts ice cream, milkshakes	low-fat frozen yogurt, sherbets, frozen fruit ices *Note:* Don't keep these frozen desserts items at home. If you are out for dinner and everyone else is having a rich dessert, choose one of these instead.
4. Bars chocolate bars	licorice, jujubes, raisins, gumdrops, jelly beans, nutritional bars such as low-fat granola or nut-seed bars *Note:* Buy these substitutions only as needed during the day so they are not in your home in large quantities to tempt you late at night. The best snack to have in the cupboard is low-fat popcorn.

What Happens in Real Life

When we are stressed, upset, or just tired, we respond by overeating or eating foods we know we should not. Identifying the problem is the first step and then understanding that between the stimulus and the response, there's an all-important gap—a chance to make a better decision. Imagine that you are walking down a cafeteria line selecting healthy food, perhaps a stir-fry and a decaffeinated drink. At the end of the line you see a slice of raspberry cheesecake. An inner voice says, "Wait a minute now. You're on this wellness program, eating only low-fat food. You're exercising every day. That cheesecake is not who you are." Another part of your brain replies, "So what; you're not going to live forever. You've had a tough morning. Enjoy yourself. It's only a little piece of cake." Anxiety, conflict, and tension move you towards the cheesecake. You say, "I'm going to hate myself later," but you do pick it up any-way. Afterwards, you berate yourself: "I can't believe I did that. I was being so good, and now I'm so bad."

There's another script you can follow instead. From now on, try this in the moment of temptation:

- Step back and visualize the saturated fat in that cheesecake entering your fat cells and making them larger, raising your blood cholesterol levels and clogging your heart and vascular system.

- Take a deep breath. Slow breathing defuses the anxiety and the craving.

- Play a game of "Let's Make a Deal." Use the gap between temptation and action to say, "I know I'm tempted, but I'm going to do something less harmful than I was about to do. It may not be the healthiest thing, but a muffin will be less harmful. And then, if I still want the raspberry cheesecake, I'll go back and have it." Don't tell yourself you will never enjoy a particular food again; you don't need that kind of pressure. Instead, on a moment-by-moment basis, start making better solution-substitution choices. Soon it will feel natural and automatic.

Joey's Turnaround

Several years ago, my friend Joey broke up with a girl he was living with. He was sad and didn't have any place to turn. I asked him if he would like to live with me for a few months until he found a new place and got his life back on track. I set three conditions: there would be no smoking, we would eat wholesome food, and we would go to the gym every day. Joey agreed and moved in.

Joey was 40 pounds overweight when our arrangement was struck and I thought this would be the ideal opportunity to get him into shape, to restore his confidence. He began with a gentle aerobic program and followed my lead at meal times. We spent many late evenings together, munching low-fat, air-popped popcorn while watching reruns of *Perry Mason*. Every morning Joey would get on the Stair Master for at least 30 minutes. Since he didn't like to push himself too hard, he stayed in the lower end of his aerobic training zone. After three months, Joey found that he had lost 36 pounds. What had changed? He'd cut out high-fat foods—no sausages, meatballs, chicken fingers, or butter on his bagels. He focused on healthier carbohydrates and he exercised for at least 30 minutes daily. Occasionally he ate some solution-substitution carbohydrates too—jujubes, licorice, and the late-night popcorn snacks. Joey didn't deprive himself completely nor did he struggle with an unrealistic diet plan. Instead, he slowly changed his relationship with food and exercise. As he progressed, he felt healthy, not hungry. He found solutions that worked for him.

Mrs L.'s Choices

Mrs. L. was a busy real estate agent. On her travels around town, she was in the habit of stopping at coffee-and-doughnut shops for a quick break. Trying to reduce her fat intake, she always intended to limit herself to black coffee, but the aroma of freshly baked doughnuts was irresistible. Always eating on the run, she found herself succumbing two or three times a day.

After working with her for several weeks, I persuaded her to break the pattern. Instead of a doughnut, she would choose a bran muffin. To keep the calories down, she would only eat the top half of the muffin—her favorite part. With one simple substitution, Mrs. L. eliminated doughnuts from her daily routine. She learned to step back and make a less damaging choice that still satisfied her craving. It would be better if she stopped drinking coffee and eating muffins altogether, but until she's ready to make that change, she substitutes a healthier alternative. The pyramids in Egypt were built of individual blocks of stone; similarly, Mrs. L. has added one more block to the structure of her new life.

The Evolution of the New You

The Two Staple Nutrition System plan represents a goal that you're working toward, and in time, you will be able to follow it almost flawlessly. But don't expect to be perfect every moment. This is not an all-or-nothing process: it's the gradual development of a wellness-oriented lifestyle.

Most individuals begin this program attached to an old habit that may be hard to break in the beginning: bacon and eggs on Sunday morning; cheddar cheese melting over a plate of nachos after a baseball game; potato chips and sour cream dip in front of the television. These are small addictions that you must overcome if you want to reduce your risk of serious disease and have the body you are shooting for.

Be prepared for the occasional setback. You may stumble sometimes on the road to success, but don't be too hard on yourself. Like Mrs. L., keep trying to make choices that are health-promoting, rather than health-hazardous. Like Joey, know that your relationship with food and exercise can change for the better.

Do your best day by day and you'll be thrilled at the results: a healthy, fit, toned, body that is younger-looking to others and to yourself.

However, there are no short cuts. That means that you must follow the Two Staple Nutrition System as I have outlined it, take the three lifelong daily supplements you learned about in Step 2 and adhere to your exercise program five to seven times per week.

Record Your Food Intake and Exercise Activity

"Record makers are record breakers" is a motto worth remembering. To kick start your program, it's helpful to record your food intake and exercise activity every day. Keep a Daily Food, Fiber, and Exercise Journal, similar to the one found in Appendix 2. You will find it much harder to cheat when you have to record your transgressions in black and white, and itemizing daily food intake and activities will give you a sense of control over the process and commitment to the program. Experience with my own patients suggests that you will greatly increase your chance of success by using a journal to help establish the habits that will eventually become second nature to you.

Adapt Your Recipes

Now that you understand the rules, you can decide whether a particular recipe or menu meets the requirements of your program. If it doesn't, you may be able to adapt it with a few simple techniques:

- Cut back, by as much as half, the amount of fat that a recipe calls for, especially the amount of oil needed to sauté vegetables.
- Thicken sauces and soups with mashed potatoes, pureed beans, or cornstarch dissolved in water.
- Instead of sautéing onions before adding them to the recipe, chop and cook them in the microwave for about 30 seconds.
- Replace all butter with olive or peanut oil.
- Substitute yogurt for sour cream or mayonnaise.
- Substitute skinned chicken for beef or pork.
- For muffins or quick breads, substitute applesauce for the same amount of oil or butter. The results will still be moist and delicious.
- Substitute two egg whites for each whole egg in a recipe.
- Use evaporated skim milk instead of cream in sauces and desserts.

Consult the Food Preparation Guide (Appendix 3) for suggestions on choosing, preparing, and serving the items recommended in the Two Staple Nutrition System.

Seven Days on the Two Staple Nutrition System

Here are seven days of sample menus using some very basic meal ideas.

DAY ONE

Breakfast	Fiber Points
whey protein shake:	
4 ounces of water, 2 ounces of orange juice, ice cubes, and 2 tablespoons of flaxseed powder mixed in a blender	1.5

Snack	
$^1/_2$ to 1 low fat bran muffin or oatmeal muffin	1.5

Lunch	
grilled chicken sandwich with vegetable toppings	0.5
minestrone soup	1.0
soda water with lemon	

Dinner	
grilled salmon	
cooked spinach	2.5
$^1/_2$ cup any bean salad with oil and vinegar dressing	2.0
diet soft drink	

Snack	
3 cups popcorn	1.5
Total	**10.5 pts**

DAY TWO

Breakfast	Fiber Points
8-10 oz. low-fat yogurt	
slice 1 nectarine and add it to yogurt	1.0
add $1/2$ cup high-fiber cereal to yogurt	
add 2 tablespoons of flaxseed powder	5.0
herbal tea	

Lunch	
1 tin of water packed tuna	
mixed green salad with oil and vinegar dressing	1.0
whole wheat roll	1.0
mineral water	

Snack	
2 plums	1.0

Dinner	
$1/4$ to $1/2$ roast chicken	
$1/2$ cup brown rice (boiled)	2.0
cranberry juice, diluted with water	

Snack	
3 cups of popcorn	1.5

Total	**12.5 pts**

DAY THREE

Breakfast	Fiber Points
1 pumpernickel bagel	1.0
3 ounces of low-fat cheese	
(e.g., creamed cottage cheese)	
1 cup sliced cantaloupe	0.5
diluted juice with two tablespoons of flaxseed powder	1.5

Snack	
1 apple	1.0

Lunch	
1 small tin salmon (water packed)	
2 slices whole wheat bread	2.0
1 sliced tomato	0.5
vegetable soup	1.0

Dinner	
4 ounces of cooked turkey breast	
mixed green salad	1.0
whole wheat roll	0.5
soda water	

Snack	
3 cups popcorn	1.5

Total	**10.5 pts**

DAY FOUR

Breakfast	Fiber Points
egg white omelette with green peppers, tomatoes, onions, and mushrooms	1.5
1 slice whole wheat toast	1.0
diluted fruit juice with two tablespoons of flaxseed powder	1.5

Lunch	
sliced turkey sandwich on a whole wheat bun, with vegetable toppings	1.0
spring water	

Snack	
two peaches	2.0

Dinner	
Pasta primavera with added chicken	1.5
mixed green salad with oil and vinegar dressing	1.0
green tea	

Snack	
Small fruit salad	1.5

Total	**11.0 pts**

DAY FIVE

Breakfast	Fiber Points
8-10 oz. low-fat plain yogurt	
add $^1/_2$ cup fresh fruit	1.0
add $^1/_2$ cup high-fiber cereal to yogurt	
and 2 tablespoons of flaxseed powder	5.0
green tea	

Lunch	
1 tin of water-packed tuna	
mixed green salad with oil and vinegar dressing	1.0
1 dinner roll	0.5
mineral water	

Snack	
1 apple	1.0

Dinner	
poached salmon in rosé wine	
steamed rice	0.75
cooked carrots	1.0
1 slice whole wheat bread (plain)	1.0
spring water	

Total	11.25 pts

DAY SIX

Breakfast	Fiber Points
whey protein shake	
(see Day One for ingredients)	1.5

Snack	
2 high-fiber biscuits	1.0
1 nectarine	1.0

Lunch	
sliced turkey breast	
pumpernickel bagel	1.0
small fruit salad	1.5
black coffee	

Dinner	
BBQ chicken	
mushrooms, artichoke hearts, tomatoes	2.0
mineral water	

Snack	
3 cups of popcorn	1.5

Total	**9.5 pts**

DAY SEVEN

Breakfast	Fiber Points
3 oz. low-fat cheese melted over an open-faced bagel	1.0
1 grapefruit	0.5
diluted juice with two tablespoons of flaxseed powder	1.5

Lunch	
sliced turkey breast	
2 slices whole wheat bread	2.0
tomatoes, lettuce	1.0
vegetable soup	1.0
mineral water	

Snack	
2 plums	1.0

Dinner	
Roasted chicken breast	
boiled rice ($^1/_2$ cup)	2.0
fruit salad (2 cups)	2.0
diet drink	

Total	**12.0 pts**

Dining Out

When you are dining away from home, it can be more difficult to stay within your guidelines. The following suggestions will help you enjoy the dining-out experience without feeling guilty.

- Ask that if possible your meal be prepared with less fat than the chef would typically use. For example, can the chef reduce the amount of oil used for stir-frying.

- When travelling by air, call ahead to request a low-fat meal or the vegetarian option.
- Salad bars are filled with high-fat extras, such as bacon bits, egg yolks, olives, and potato salads. Bypass these foods in favour of fresh vegetables. Ask for sauces and dressings to be served on the side. This way you can control how much you use.
- Order baked potatoes, rice, or pasta instead of French fries.
- Order plain bean tostadas or bean burritos.
- Order fish or chicken sandwiches without the sauce. Make sure they are grilled, not fried.

Chinese Restaurants

- A personal favorite is Moo Goo Gai Pan, a bed of steamed rice covered with stir-fried vegetables—broccoli, onions, Swiss chard, Chinese vegetables, carrots, and shrimp or chicken.
- You might also want to try:

  -vegetable chow mein or chop suey

  -orange chicken

  -shrimp in garlic or tomato sauce
- Avoid fried dishes, especially foods in batter (such as chicken balls or lemon chicken), and pork selections.

Italian Restaurants

- As an appetizer, try:

  -minestrone soup

  -radicchio salad, dressing on the side

  -grilled calamari salad, oil dressing on the side.

- For the main course, consider:
  -pasta primavera, add chicken
  -pasta with seafood in a red sauce
  -any grilled fish or chicken.

Mexican Restaurants

- A popular choice is chicken fajitas, made with stir-fried chicken and onion. Make a sandwich by rolling chicken, onions, and other vegetables with salsa in a soft tortilla. Leave out the sour cream and guacamole, both of which are high in fat.
- Bean burritos are also quite low in fat, if you forego the cheese.

Chicken Restaurants

Good choices include:
- Chicken breast, grilled or barbecued with skin removed.
- Baked potato or rice; no French fries. Eat the potato without the butter or margarine.
- Whole wheat roll, no butter.

Deli Restaurants

- Turkey sandwich on whole wheat, pumpernickel, or rye bread with tomato, lettuce, and mustard for moisture, but no butter, margarine, or mayonnaise.
- Chicken breast sandwich.
- Single serving of canned salmon or tuna on a plate, no mayonnaise.
- Toasted bagel or bread, no butter or margarine.

- Mixed salad, dressing on the side.

- Vegetable, pea, or minestrone soup.

- Pancakes occasionally, instead of waffles or bacon and eggs. Use just a little syrup, but no butter. Buckwheat pancakes are the healthiest choice.

Fast-Food Restaurants

- Try the salad bar or grilled or barbecued chicken.

The Intensive Weight Loss Plan

For those of you who are overweight, I have created an intensive phase weight loss plan using the principles of the Two Staple Nutrition System. This is a highly structured program that will ensure the weight loss results that are important in terms of self-image and overall wellness. As we've seen, being overweight significantly increases your risk of heart attack, stroke, high blood pressure, gallbladder disease, adult onset diabetes, breast cancer, osteoarthritis, and possibly prostate and colon cancer.

This version of the Two Staple Nutrition System will enable you to lose weight without slowing down your metabolism, as is often the case with very low-calorie diets and many high protein diets. Such diets can put your body into a state of ketosis, in which the weight loss is the result of a breakdown of lean muscle tissue. With loss of your lean mass, your metabolism slows down dramatically. To avoid regaining weight, you will have to stay on a calorie-restricted program for the rest of your life, forever refusing pasta, rice, bread, and potatoes. By contrast, my intensive weight loss plan will enable you to lose fat while maintaining or increasing lean mass and metabolic rate. You will look and feel vibrant and, once down to your ideal weight, you will keep the pounds off while enjoying a full range of healthy foods for the rest of your life.

As with the Two Staple System, record the foods you eat, the fiber you consume, the supplements you take and the physical activity you perform in a Daily Food, Fiber, and Exercise Journal. This type of self-monitoring has been shown to be a powerful incentive to long-term weight loss success.

The Intensive Weight Loss Plan provides 1,200 to 1,500 calories per day. In conjunction with the prescribed minimum amount of daily physical activity—a 30 minute power walk—most individuals will lose two pounds a week. Fluctuations in body water and other factors may prevent weight loss from occurring in a consistent manner from week to week, but over the first five-week period a 10-pound loss of body fat is normal.

This diet is moderately high in protein, low in fat, and provides safe and adequate levels of mostly Category 1, 2, and 3 carbohydrates, plus vitamins and minerals. Proportionately; it comprises approximately 50 percent carbohydrates, 30 percent protein and 20 percent fat.

THREE MEALS PLUS THREE SNACKS PER DAY	
Breakfast:	1 high-protein breakfast selection
Mid-morning Snack:	1 fruit selection
Lunch:	1 flesh protein selection
	1 vegetable selection
	1-2 bread selections*
Afternoon Snack:	1 fruit selection
Dinner:	1 flesh protein selection
	1 vegetable selection
	1-2 bread selections*
Evening Snack:	3-6 cups of low-fat popcorn
	No butter is allowed; use margarine sparingly or not at all. Avoid juices, jams, and jellies.

*One serving of pasta, rice, or potatoes may be substituted for two bread servings.

Other Daily Requirements:

1. 6-8 (8-oz.) glasses of fluids per day;

2. High-potency multiple vitamin and mineral;

3. Fat Burner supplement: one caplet taken at lunch and dinner;

4. Minimum 30-minute power-walk or aerobic program of your choice. Resistance training in addition will help increase your lean mass and resting metabolic rate.

High-Protein Breakfast Selections

1. Egg white omelette (3 or 4 egg whites) with $1/2$ cup of desired vegetables (no butter or margarine, use a small amount of olive oil)

   1 sliced tomato

2. Egg Beaters—1 serving size with $1/2$ cup of vegetables

3. Protein shake—1 serving of protein powder shake mix (providing 20-25 grams of whey, egg white, or soy protein, no more that 6 grams of carbohydrates and less than 2 grams of fat), mixed in a blender with 4-6 ounces of cold water, ice cubes, and 2 tablespoons of flaxseed powder.

4. 8 oz non-fat sugarless yogurt and $1/3$ cup cereal *or* 1% milk or skim milk and cereal

   Appropriate cereals:

100% Bran	Wheetabix
All-Bran	Raw Oatmeal
Bran Buds	Puffed Wheat
Bran Flakes	Shredded Wheat

Fiber 1   Nabisco 100% Bran Cereal

Grape Nuts   Special K

Any other unsweetened cereal with a high fiber content

Lunch and Dinner Selections

At both lunch and dinner, the same formula applies:

- 1 Flesh Protein Selection (for example, chicken breast)
- 1 Vegetable Selection (e.g., a bowl of minestrone soup)
- 1 or 2 Bread Selections (1 or 2 pieces of dry toast)

Three bread servings are permitted each day. If you have two at lunch, then you must have only one for dinner and vice versa. If you have cereal for breakfast you are permitted only two bread servings for the remainder of that day.

1 bread serving equals one of the following:

- 1 slice of bread
- $\frac{1}{2}$ bagel
- 4 soda crackers
- 2 pieces of melba toast
- 2 rice cracker biscuits (unsweetened)
- $\frac{1}{2}$ of a 4" x 6" matzoh
- $\frac{1}{2}$ kaiser bun
- $\frac{1}{2}$ English muffin
- 1 small dinner roll

One serving of pasta, rice, or potatoes counts as two bread servings and maybe substituted for bread occasionally. All are easily converted into fat, however, so have no more than two selections from this food group per week (for example 1 pasta selection and

1 rice selection = 2 selections).

One serving size equals one of the following:

- pasta: 1 cup cooked with tomato sauce
- rice: 1 cup cooked (boiled, steamed)
- potatoes: 1 whole potato (baked or boiled)

Beverages

Every day, you should drink six to eight glasses of water. Distilled water, spring water, low-sodium mineral water, and soda water are all good choices. Drink two glasses before each meal. Bottled water should be ozone-treated to help prevent bacterial growth. The best water is either distilled or has undergone reverse osmosis and deionization.

Keep your intake of caffeinated beverages to a minimum, at no more than three cups of coffee or tea a day. It's best to drink them black, but if you can't, use non-fat or 1% low-fat milk and artificial sweeteners. Try herbal teas or hot water and lemon as an alternative to coffee or regular tea. Green tea is an excellent substitute.

Diet drinks that contain aspartame are the most acceptable soft drinks, but don't overdo it: two servings maximum per day. Avoid all beverages sweetened with sugar and beware of high-sodium drinks. They make your body retain sodium and water, creating a bloated sensation.

Oils and Salad Dressings

The preferred oils are olive oil, peanut oil, and canola oil. Use the least amount possible (1 tsp. for every 1 serving size) for a stir-fry, to sauté vegetables, to brown meats, in tomato sauces or for salad dressings. Salad dressings should be made from olive oil and vinegar, or use 1 tsp of a low-fat Italian dressing.

Food Selections and One-Serving Sizes

Low-Fat Flesh Protein Selections:

One serving of chicken, turkey, Cornish hen, fish, tofu products: 3-4 ounces.

Vegetable Selections:

Option 1

One serving size is up to 3 cups of the following vegetables in a salad:

- carrots
- peppers
- dark green leafy vegetables
- tomatoes
- broccoli
- cauliflower
- onions
- cucumbers
- radicchio

Option 2

A serving is one of the following items:

- $1/2$ cup cooked carrots
- $1/2$ cup of raw or cooked broccoli, cauliflower, Brussels sprouts or cabbage
- $1/2$ cup of cooked spinach or other greens such as bok choy or rapini
- $1/2$ cup of cooked zucchini

- $^3/_4$ cup of cooked peppers
- $^1/_2$ cup of beets
- $^1/_2$ cup of cooked asparagus
- $^1/_3$ cup of cooked corn
- 1 ear of corn on the cob
- $^1/_2$ cup of beans, peas, or lentils (cooked or dried)

Option 3

A serving is one bowl of soup (non-cream, non-milk, non-chowder)—vegetable, minestrone, or pea soup (no ham).

Fruits

A serving is one of the following:

- 1 apple
- 2 apricots
- $^1/_2$ banana
- $^1/_2$ cup of berries
- $^1/_2$ cup of cantaloupe
- 10 large cherries
- 2 dates
- 1 fig
- $^1/_2$ grapefruit
- 12 grapes
- $^1/_3$ honeydew melon
- $^1/_2$ mango
- 1 nectarine
- 1 orange
- $^3/_4$ cup of papaya

- 1 peach
- 1 pear
- 1 persimmon
- $1/4$ cup of pineapple
- 2 plums
- 2 prunes
- 2 tbsp. of raisins
- 1 tangerine
- 1 cup of watermelon

Potato

A serving is one potato with no butter. You may use low-calorie margarine, but no sour cream unless it is non-fat.

Dairy

A serving is one of the following:

- 1 cup (8 oz.) skim or non-fat milk
- 1 cup (8 oz.) yogurt made from skim milk or
- 1% milk (plain, or sweetened without sugar or fruit)
- $1/4$ cup (2 oz.) soy cheese or other cheese (less than 4% milk fat or total fat)
- 2-3 oz. low-fat cottage cheese (not creamed)
- 3-4 egg whites (no yolks allowed)

Seasonings

All spices and herbs are allowed except those which are sodium-based or which contain sodium. Celery salt, garlic salt, and onion salt, for example, are not allowed.

Allowable seasonings:

Aspartame	Mustard
Basil	Nutmeg
Celery seasoning	Onion Powder
Cinnamon	Oregano
Cumin	Parsley
Garlic	Pepper
Lemon	Pepper
Lemon	Rosemary
Morton's salt	Vinegar

A Typical Day on the Intensive Weight Loss Plan

Breakfast

3-egg-white omelette with mushrooms, green peppers, and onions served with sliced tomatoes

1 cup of black coffee with sweetener

Midmorning Snack

1 nectarine

soda water

Lunch

broiled skinless chicken breast

bowl of vegetable soup

1 dinner roll

1 diet cola

Afternoon Snack

$^{1}/_{2}$ cup cantaloupe slices

mineral water

(continued)

(Continued)

Dinner

4 oz. grilled swordfish

one large mixed salad with olive oil and vinegar dressing

spring water

Evening Snack

3-6 cups of low-fat microwave popcorn

2-3 glasses of soda water

Multivitamin and Mineral Supplement

Exercise

30-minute power walk after dinner

Fat Burner Supplement

3 capsules

Fat Burning Supplements Can Speed Weight Loss

It's well established that some people gain weight more easily and have more difficulty losing weight than others. Animal research and human twin studies reveal that genetic factors may play a role in susceptibility to weight gain. In the past decade, a number of intervention trials with overweight subjects have investigated responses to this phenomenon. They have found that three naturally occurring nutrients, when taken at optimal doses, can facilitate weight loss, even in subjects with a genetic predisposition to weight problems.

These three metabolic fat-burning conditioning agents help the body overcome the resistance to fat-burning that is frequently encountered in overweight individuals. In conjunction with the Two Staple Nutrition System and exercise, they can help speed up metabolism, enabling the body to burn more calories while at rest.

Unlike ephedra, an herbal product that can adversely affect the heart and nervous system, these nutrients are completely safe and produce no undesirable side effects at recommended levels of intake. The fat-burning trio of metabolic conditioners I am referring to are chromium, hydroxycitric acid (HCA), and coleus forskohlii.

Chromium: Blocking the Conversion of Carbohydrate to Fat

One of the most frustrating aspects of being overweight is that your body tends to convert carbohydrates into fat with greater ease. As body fat increases, the cells become less sensitive to the effects of the hormone insulin. The pancreas must secrete ever-higher levels of insulin to overcome the body's insulin resistance. As we know, insulin is needed to help the cells extract glucose from the blood-stream. But higher levels of insulin encourage the liver to convert more carbohydrates into fat following a meal or snack containing carbohydrate foods. The newly formed fats are shipped to your fat cells, contributing to further weight gain and increased body fat. It becomes a vicious cycle—and a low-fat diet alone won't help, because your body is conditioned to convert carbohydrates into fat by its high levels of circulating insulin.

Insulin requires the presence of the mineral chromium in order to maximize its effect on body tissue. Studies have demonstrated that when subjects supplemented with chromium, their body tissues became much more sensitive to the influence of insulin and the amount of insulin secreted was significantly reduced. Most diets contain only 25 to 50 micrograms of chromium per day. To optimize insulin sensitivity, levels of 200 to 400 mcg are required. Only through supplementation is it possible to ensure chromium intake in this range.

Endurance exercise also helps to increase insulin sensitivity and lower circulating insulin levels. Thus, regular exercise and chromium supplementation are a powerful combination in body fat reduction and insulin regulation.

Chromium and exercise can also increase your metabolism, speeding up the rate at which your body burns fuels at rest. By aiding the action of insulin, chromium helps to increase the delivery of protein to your muscles. If you exercise regularly, more protein gets laid down inside the muscle, increasing muscle tone, definition, and lean mass. As your lean mass increases, your body burns more calories every minute, since muscles burn calories even at rest. As a result your metabolism speeds up, allowing you to eat more calories without gaining weight.

Together, regular exercise and chromium supplementation help block the conversion of carbohydrates into fat and facilitate an increase in lean mass, tone, definition, and metabolism. Studies using chromium supplementation have confirmed its effects on body fat reduction and increases in lean mass.

Hydroxycitric Acid (HCA): A Natural Appetite Suppressant with No Side Effects

Another effective metabolic conditioner that aids in weight loss is hydroxycitric acid (HCA), a naturally occurring appetite suppressant that is found in the rind of the garcinia cambogia fruit. Traditionally, it has been used as a food additive and condiment in many dishes native to the Southeast Asian countries in which it grows. Toxicity studies have shown that HCA is an extremely safe dietary supplement, with no reported toxicity at recommended intake levels. A the same time, studies on human subjects have demonstrated remarkable weight loss results at doses of 750 mg to 1500 mg.

The available research indicates that HCA inhibits the key enzymes that convert carbohydrates into fat. As a result, the liver shunts carbohydrates to its carbohydrate fuel tank. As the tank fills, nerve signals travel from the liver to the brain that suppress appetite. Simply stated, you feel content and stuffed. HCA offers a double benefit: it blocks the conversion of carbohydrate into fat and it triggers nerve signals that suppress appetite, thus reducing the tendency to overeat.

Best of all, appetite suppression occurs in a natural way. Drugs like ephedra are known to have life-threatening side effects, acting directly on the central nervous system.

Some studies involving subjects taking 750 mg of HCA per day have demonstrated weight losses in subjects of almost 20 pounds in just eight weeks, even in patients who had reached a weight loss plateau on a prior two-month diet plan.

Coleus Forskohlii

Coleus forskohlii is a member of the mint family and is recognized in the world of herbal medicine as the only plant source of the diterpene compound known as forskolin. What makes forskolin so important is its ability to stimulate the synthesis of cyclic adenosine monophosphate (AMP), which among other outcomes, triggers the release of fat from fat cells and speeds up metabolism by increasing the rate at which the body burns calories at rest. Another agent known to produce a similar effect is ephedrine and its adrenaline-like sister compounds, all capable of dangerous side effects. Unlike ephedrine, forskolin does not stimulate the nervous system. Clinical trials involving overweight human subjects have demonstrated that supplementation with a standardized grade of coleus forskohlii can help patients lose up to 10 pounds in just eight weeks. Subjects also increased their lean mass, which further speeds up the resting metabolic rate.

Experimental evidence suggests that forskolin may also have a mild thyroid stimulating action, which may also explain its effectiveness in helping overweight subjects increase their metabolism and thermogenic activity. However, more research is required to determine if forskolin affects the thyroid gland in living subjects in a similar manner as it does in laboratory studies. My experience indicates that the combination of chromium, hydroxycitric acid and coleus forskohlii, taken as an adjunct to a proper weight management program, can be quite useful.

Together with a proper nutrition and lifestyle plan, these three ingredients have been shown to be safe and effective. I routinely recommend the inclusion of a dietary supplement containing these three metabolic fat-burning conditioning agents to my weight loss patients and to other health practitioners. The product I prefer contains the following in a single capsule: chromium – 66.7 mcg; hydroxycitric acid – 333.4 mg; coleus forskolin – 66.7 mg.

I suggest one or two capsules, three times a day with meals, during the weight reduction period. A maintenance dose of two or three capsules daily can help maintain weight loss indefinitely and improve blood sugar regulation for individuals with non-insulin dependent diabetes, glucose intolerance, or syndrome X, a pre-diabetic state.

Starting Right Now...

1. Buy a notebook or loose leaf binder and set up your Daily Food, Fiber, and Exercise Journal. Tomorrow morning, start making your entries. Even if you are not yet on a full exercise and eating program, these early entries will focus your mind on the changes you want to make.

2. Prepare a shopping list of the food items that are included in the Two Staple Nutrition System and stockpile them in your home. That way, you'll always have the right foods on hand.

3. Go through your favorite recipes and adapt them to your new wellness lifestyle. Toss out those you can't adapt; if you don't have them, you won't use them.

4. Purchase or borrow a few wellness-oriented cookbooks and add new recipes to your repertoire. Start a file of healthy recipes clipped from magazines and newspapers.

5. Enlist your spouse or family in the effort: tell them your plan for healthy eating and ask for their help. Better yet, ask them to join you.

For access to the references to Step 4 and additional education on wellness please visit the author's web site at www.renaisante.com

STEP 5

Anti-Aging Supplements After Age 40

Although we may pride ourselves on having evolved spiritually, intellectually, and emotionally, as a species we have not evolved very far biologically. After the age of forty, our bodies are programmed to start aging: parts wear out, tissues break down, and we become increasingly vulnerable to life-threatening diseases and infections. Embedded in our genes are the blueprints for age-related changes that will prompt our physiological features to decline and degenerate, leading ultimately to our demise.

Why do our bodies allow this to happen? Because as far as nature is concerned, once we have lived long enough to reproduce and foster the next generation, we have served our biological purpose on this planet. After that, we are taking up precious space, eating valuable food, consuming a lot of oxygen, and creating too much waste. Nature has equipped each of us with an exit strategy from the day of conception, and its highlights include crippling arthritis, loss of muscle and bone mass leading to osteoporotic fractures, angina, heart disease, congestive heart failure, virulent infections, brain degeneration with memory loss, dementia and Alzheimer's disease, macular degeneration of the eye, cataracts, and cancer.

For years it was assumed that these end-game conditions were inevitable, that there was little to be done to prevent or postpone their development. Today, however, the evidence argues against this deterministic viewpoint. Science has identified many of the body's clockwork-like biological adjustments, those changes that are designed to initiate deterioration. We now know that the body can accelerate the aging process and increase our risk of disease by trigging a decline or rise in the synthesis or secretion of certain hormones, a decline or rise in the strength of certain enzymes, and by gradually allowing the immune system to weaken. These are the primary alterations that occur automatically in the body after the age of 40. A healthy diet and exercise alone are not enough to forestall their arrival or counter their effects.

Fortunately, virtually all of these age-related changes can be influenced by the use of targeted, natural, anti-aging nutritional supplements. A comprehensive program that incorporates nutrition and exercise plus supplementation can compensate for the body's midlife reprogramming, slow biological aging, and significantly reduce your vulnerability to the degenerative aliments associated with old age. It's not necessary to accept the common discomforts of old age; there is something you can do about them.

The resilient nature of the human body is now beginning to be appreciated. Breakthrough discoveries in anti-aging and disease prevention are being made just at a time when baby boomers and young seniors are moving into their high-risk years. Many are already committed to taking proactive measures to remain healthy as long as possible and to avoid or postpone the degenerative diseases that their parents and grandparents suffered. Convinced of the benefits of nutritional supplements, they have helped drive annual sales to $2 billion a year in Canada and $16 billion a year in the United States. Surveys indicate that 60 to 70 percent of North American adults use nutritional supplements on a regular basis. The only issue for these motivated individuals is to know which supplements most effectively contribute to anti-aging and disease prevention.

Unfortunately, some members of the medical profession are either unaware of or have chosen to ignore the burgeoning research in this area. They remain focused on a reductionist model of health delivery, providing a single remedy—usually a synthetic drug—for a single condition and treating symptoms rather than underlying causes. However, a growing number of medical doctors who belong to the American College for the Advancement of Medicine and the Academy of Anti-Aging Research hold a different view. They are strong proponents of the use of supplements and other cutting edge interventions to inhibit and reverse the biological process of aging.

Through published studies and experimental trials, ten specific supplement interventions have been shown to be highly effective. In the pages following, we'll examine the science behind these important anti-aging supplements. In my view, you should incorporate all into your lifetime wellness program after age 40: you will slow the aging process, reduce the risk of degenerative diseases, and enhance your appearance, feelings of wellbeing, and quality of life as you age.

1. Coenzyme Q10 and the Heart, Brain, and Immune System—and Cancer Prevention

Coenzyme Q10 (CoQ10), also known as ubiquinone, is a vitamin-like substance that is required for the production of energy in every cell of your body. In order to survive and carry out their specialized functions, cells must continually convert some of the food you eat into a usable source of energy called adenosine triphosphate (ATP-energy). CoQ10 enables your cells to make this conversion, within the mitochondria—the energy factory of the cell. If your cells cannot produce sufficient amounts of ATP-energy due to a CoQ10 deficiency, then a decline in cell function occurs that can hasten the onset of heart disease, a decline in brain function, a weakening of the immune system, and a heightened cancer risk. More recently, we have seen that CoQ10 deficiency is an underlying cause of Parkinson's disease and a contributing factor in many cases of congestive heart failure and high blood pressure.

CoQ10 Synthesis Declines as We Age

The body generates optimal amounts of CoQ10 up to about age 20. After that, a decline in CoQ10 synthesis begins, becoming significant around age 40. The natural synthesis of CoQ10 is a 17-step process that involves eight vitamins (mostly the B vitamins) and several minerals. Some of the enzymes required in this process disappear with age, which impairs the ability of the body to make the amount of CoQ10 it needs. The intake of CoQ10-containing foods alone is not enough to compensate. The average daily intake of CoQ10 from food is five to 10 mg. This is adequate up to a certain age, while your body is making most of what it needs. But studies suggest that 30 to 60 mg of CoQ10 supplementation a day is desirable after age 40; dosages in the range of 150 to 300 mg a day are required to favorably affect outcomes in patients with congestive heart failure, failing memory, Parkinson's disease or for cancer treatment support. You would have to consume half a pound of sardines or two and a half pounds of peanuts a day to yield 30 mg of CoQ10 intake.

Certain medications interfere with the body's ability to absorb CoQ10. If you are taking any of the following, you should ingest 30 to 60 mg a day of CoQ10 to compensate, regardless of how young or old you are:

- Orlistat: Don't take CoQ10 supplements within 90 minutes of ingesting Orlistat
- Beta blockers
- Biguanides
- Clondine

- Gemfibrozil
- Haloperidol
- HMG-CoA reductase inhibitors
- Hydralazine
- Methydopa
- Phenothiazines
- Sulfonylureas: some of these drugs decrease CoQ10 synthesis (acetohexamide, glyburide, tolazamide)
- Thiazide diuretics
- Tricyclic antidepressants

Coenzyme Q10 supplementation is a necessity by age 40 to 50. In essence, supplementation with CoQ10 allows you put the CoQ10 back into your body to compensate for what your body can no longer provide for itself. It is a safe, effective, and essential natural anti-aging intervention that counters the body's aging.

Congestive Heart Failure and CoQ10

A decline in CoQ10 levels has been shown to contribute to the development of congestive heart failure, a condition in which the heart muscle becomes too weak to pump blood through the arteries and blood vessels. More specifically, a lack of CoQ10 prevents the heart muscle from producing the ATP energy it requires to contract with enough force to pump blood through the system. As a result, blood circulation backs up and fluid leaks out of the blood vessels into the lungs, the hands and the feet, which leads to shortness of breath, swelling of the extremities, and high blood pressure. Biopsy and blood sample results from the hearts of patients with various age-related cardiovascular diseases, especially congestive heart failure, show a deficiency in CoQ10 in 50 to 75 percent of subjects.

Several well-designed clinical studies have demonstrated that CoQ10 supplementation can reverse congestive heart failure in a significant number of cases enabling the heart muscle to once again produce the ATP energy it requires. Discontinuation resulted in severe relapses of congestive heart failure in research subjects. In cases such as these, CoQ10 supplementation must be a lifelong strategy. The beneficial effects of CoQ10 supplementation may not be evident for several months, while CoQ10 concentrations build up in the heart muscle. Generally speaking, CoQ10 can be taken with other drugs that are used to treat congestive heart failure, high blood pressure, or other heart ailments, and studies show that its use often allows doctors to reduce the number of medications required to control these conditions. However, if you are currently suffering from congestive heart failure or any other heart condition or high blood pressure, you should do not undertake CoQ10 supplementation without first notifying your doctor.

As surprising as it may seem, most doctors and cardiologists in the United States and Canada do not prescribe CoQ10 supplementation as part of their usual treatment protocols for heart conditions. This is largely due to the influence of drug companies. CoQ10 cannot be patented as a drug, so it does not represent a source of profits for drug companies. However, CoQ10 supplementation is widely prescribed for the treatment of congestive heart failure and other cardiovascular conditions by doctors in Italy, Sweden, Israel, and Japan, who report significant improvement in a high percentage of their patients. In fact, many individuals in these countries take CoQ10 supplementation for prevention as well as for therapeutic purposes: 15 percent of Swedes and 20 percent of Danes take CoQ10 supplements, according to one survey. As far back as 1987, there were more than 10 million citizens in Japan using CoQ10 supplementation for the treatment of heart-related conditions.

In many cases, congestive heart failure appears to be caused by the age-related decline in CoQ10 synthesis that is programmed into our genes. It makes sense to supplement your diet with CoQ10 as a way to prevent congestive heart failure from developing in the first place. Beginning between the ages of 40 and 50 years, take at least 30 mg of CoQ10 per day. By age 60 to 65, it may be wise to increase the dosage to 60 mg per day. Patients with congestive heart failure usually require higher dosages to combat the ailment on a therapeutic level. It's not uncommon for doctors to recommend 150 to 300 mg per day, taken in divided doses (50 mg three times daily or 150 mg twice daily). A significant CoQ10 blood level, usually greater than 3.5 micrograms per milliliter, is necessary to obtain a therapeutic effect.

High Blood Pressure, and Angina, and CoQ10

Preliminary research indicates that a lack of CoQ10 synthesis may also contribute to the development of high blood pressure, angina and irregular heartbeat problems. In these cases, daily dosages in the range of 100 to 200 mg have been shown to be successful in improving exercise performance in patients suffering from angina, in lowering high blood pressure by nine to 20 percent, and in reducing the number of episodes of irregular heartbeats in patients with mitral valve prolapse. To help counter these problems, begin taking a CoQ10-containing supplement after age 40.

Preserving Brain Function with CoQ10

Recent studies have highlighted the fact that the brain has higher CoQ10 concentrations than the blood, the heart, or any other organ. Just like the heart, the brain requires CoQ10 to make the

ATP energy necessary to perform its distinctive functions. And just as with the heart, brain levels of CoQ10 decline as we age, which can contribute to impaired cognitive function. A lack of CoQ10 makes it more difficult for brain cells to manufacture the chemicals they need for clear thinking, concentration, memory recall, information processing, coordination of movement, and even to maintain balance during standing and walking. CoQ10 deficiency may also be significant to the development of degenerative brain diseases such as Lou Gehrig's disease (amyotrophic lateral sclerosis), Huntington's disease, Parkinson's disease, Alzheimer's disease and other conditions that affect the brain and nervous system. In addition, CoQ10 is an important brain antioxidant, known to protect brain cells from the free radicals that are strongly associated with most brain degenerative diseases. The brain uses at least 10 percent of the body's oxygen at any given moment, a side effect of which is the creation of many oxygen free radicals, a natural if potentially harmful consequence of oxygen metabolism, as we saw in Step 2 of this book. Antioxidants such as vitamin E and vitamin C have been shown to concentrate in the brain and protect brain tissue from free radical damage, but recent studies have established that CoQ10 is also an essential brain antioxidant. Along with other antioxidants, CoQ10 supplementation is one of the best anti-aging interventions you can adopt to preserve brain function and help guard against degenerative disorders.

Parkinson's Disease and CoQ10

In the past few years a number of researchers have concluded that a significant cause of Parkinson's disease is a genetic inability to synthesize adequate amounts of CoQ10 in parts of the brain affected by the disease. They suggest that supplementation with CoQ10 can compensate for this defect and potentially prevent the disease onset or further progression. In the October 2002 issue of

Archives of Neurology, Dr. Clifford Shults and fellow researchers presented the findings of a clinical trial demonstrating that patients with early-stage Parkinson's disease who were given CoQ10 supplementation for 16 months showed significantly less impairment than did patients given the placebo. The efficacy of treatment was readily apparent by the eight-month mark: those patients given the highest doses of CoQ10 had the best overall results. The test doses were 300, 600, and 1,200 mg per day. The side effects were mostly mild and included back pain, headaches, and dizziness.

The researchers indicated that the administration of CoQ10 was aimed not only at symptomatic relief, but at the underlying biochemical disorders associated with the development of the disease, namely that individuals become prone to Parkinson's as result of not being able synthesize enough CoQ10 in critical parts of the brain. As a result, those brain cells lack the ATP energy needed to make sufficient amounts of dopamine, without which the individual suffers the disease's characteristic tremors and other involuntary movements, as well as progressive weakness. The lack of ATP energy eventually leads to the degeneration and death of many of these brain cells, which allows the condition to progress to its life-threatening end-stages.

Dr. Shults's research was the first placebo-controlled study to show that CoQ10 supplementation can halt the progression of early-stage Parkinson's disease in human subjects. It involved only 80 subjects (40 in the CoQ10 group and 40 in the placebo group), but these impressive findings have paved the way for larger studies that should more clearly establish the degree to which CoQ10 supplementation is useful as a treatment and possibly as a preventive agent in high-risk populations.

Parkinson's disease primarily afflicts individuals over the age of 50, the phase of life when most people experience a significant age-related decline in CoQ10 synthesis. Today, over one million Americans and approximately 100,000 Canadians suffer from it, but the incidence of the disease in younger people is increasing at an alarming rate, according to the American Parkinson's Disease Association.

Immune Function and CoQ10

It is well documented that the body's immune system becomes weaker and less effective as we age. This is the reason that we become prone to more serious and life-threatening infections in later years and accounts in part for the fact that cancer incidence rises with every decade of life. A well-functioning immune system helps your body kill off any potentially harmful viruses, bacteria, and other germs that can infect or alter the DNA of certain tissues, leading to cancerous mutations. Certain cells of the immune system, such as natural killer cells, actually seek out and destroy developing cancer cells before they can do damage.

Like other cells in the body, immune cells require ample CoQ10 in order to synthesize the ATP energy they need, yet the decline in CoQ10 synthesis that occurs with age results in a decline in immune function that becomes quite pronounced after the age of 50. Both animal and human studies show that CoQ10 supplementation improves immune system function in older animals and human subjects, and reverses some aspects of immune system decline. In one human study, chronically ill patients who were given 60 mg per day of CoQ10 for 27 to 98 days showed significantly increased blood levels of immu-noglobulin G (IgG), an important antibody that destroys viruses and other microbes that may cause infection.

CoQ10 and Cancer Treatment Support

CoQ10 has shown antioxidant, tumor-suppressive, and im-mune-strengthening effects in both experimental and human studies. For these reasons it is often recommended not only to help prevent cancer, but also as part of the nutrition and supplementation support program to discourage the recurrence or progression of cancer in patients who have already been afflicted.

The most convincing evidence for its application in this regard was demonstrated by a study involving 32 women with breast cancer, aged 32 to 81 years. These women were classified as high-risk for the spread of cancer because their axillary lymph nodes showed evidence of cancer cells in biopsy examination. After completing the standard radiation and chemo-therapy that followed their surgeries, the women were given high-dose nutritional supplementation: vitamin C, 2850 mg; vitamin E, 2500 IU; beta-carotene, 32.5 mg; selenium, 387 mcg; secondary vitamins and minerals; an essential fatty acid supplement consisting of 1200 mg of gamma-linolenic acid and 3500 mg of omega-3 fats (e.g., flaxseed oil), and Coenzyme Q10, 90 to 300 mg. At the end of the 18-month study none of the patients had died during the study period (the expected number of deaths derived from medical statistics was four); none experienced a further spread or metastasis of their cancer; the quality of life scores improved (no weight loss; reduced use of painkillers); and six patients showed apparent partial remission. The patients consuming the higher dosages of CoQ10 (300 mg per day) appeared to show the best results in terms of quality of life scores and partial remission.

As a result of these findings I often recommend an updated version of this supplementation program to individuals who have had cancer to enhance immune function and help suppress tumor growth.

Whether we have experienced serious age-related disease by age 40 or not, given our declining synthesis of CoQ10 it is vital to supplement with this nutrient as a means of forestalling the aging process. I recommend that you begin taking a CoQ10-containing supplement at age 40, or at the latest by age 50. If you are on medications that impair CoQ10 absorption or synthesis, or if you have any of the health conditions mentioned in this chapter, then begin taking it earlier. Remember that CoQ10 is a fat-soluble nutrient and therefore it is absorbed into your bloodstream only if you take it with meals that contain some fat. Don't take CoQ10 supplements on an empty stomach or with a piece of toast and jam; always take it with a meal. Be aware too that alpha-linolenic acid—an essential fatty acid found in flaxseed oil—has been shown to greatly enhance the absorption of CoQ10.

The final piece of information to know regarding CoQ10 supplementation is that the active ingredients in hawthorn berries and hawthorn leaves maximize the ATP energy-generating effect of CoQ10. Hawthorn (*crataegus oxyacantha*) is a spiny tree or shrub that is native to Europe. Its leaves and berries contain flavonoids compounds known as prosyanidins that provide its medicinal effects. In Japan and other Asian counties, as well as Germany and other parts of Europe, supplementation with a standardized grade of hawthorn has been shown to reverse congestive heart failure, lower blood pressure, and improve cases of angina. When taken together, CoQ10 and hawthorn optimize the production of ATP energy in many body tissues. (Patients on digitalis or digoxin should not take hawthorn without a physician's consent.)

It is important to use a standardized grade of hawthorn, which contains three to five percent flavonoid or procyanidin content, to ensure enough of its active ingredients to be effective. My preference is to take a CoQ10 supplement that also contains hawthorn, to simplify the process. In general, there should about 37.5 mg of hawthorn for every 30 mg of CoQ10 present in the supplement. This provides an ideal anti-aging synergistic effect to maximize ATP energy production in the body.

2. The "Detoxification and Immune Function Four": Milk Thistle, Indole-3-Carbinole, Reishi Mushroom Extract, and Astragalus

Part of nature's plan for the decline of our bodies after age 40 is the deterioration of detoxification enzymes in our liver cells and the disabling of our white blood cells —the very cells that identify and destroy cancer cells and fight off viruses and potentially fatal infections. This loss of detoxification capacity and immune function accounts for the rise in cancer rates in older populations. It's also the reason why someone who is 85 years of age is more likely to find himself in a life-threatening situation, if he contracts pneumonia, than would an 18-year-old. Among men, 75 percent of new cancer cases and 82 percent of cancer deaths occur after the age of 60. Women in the same age group experience 63 percent of new cases of cancer and 78 percent of cancer deaths.

All this is related in part to a faulty detoxification function (which allows carcinogens to build up in our bodies as we age), coupled with the weakening of the immune system (which impairs the ability of our immune cells—the white blood cells—to destroy cancer cells and fend off infections). It is well known that drugs like prednisone, which suppresses the body's immune system, increase cancer risk to a significant degree. It is also acknowledged that individuals with AIDS, who have compromised immune function, are extremely susceptible to the development of certain cancers. There is no doubt that a healthy immune system and the prevention of cancer go hand-in-hand.

Researchers have discovered that the use of certain nutritional supplements can boost the performance of the body's detoxification enzymes and immune. By taking a combination of these herbal agents in conjunction with the nutritional program outlined in this book and a high-potency multivitamin and mineral supplement, you can provide your body with the daily nutrient support it needs. The four herbal products to add to your list of daily anti-aging and disease preventing supplements are milk thistle, indole-3-carbinol, reishi mushroom extract, and astragalus. To understand their benefits, it's helpful to know how our detoxification and immune systems operate.

Detoxification and Nutrition

The liver is the primary site for the detoxification of carcinogens, toxins, end products of metabolism, older circulating hormones, and other food-borne environmental chemicals, such as pesticides, herbicides, and artificial food additives. Almost two quarts of blood pass through the liver every minute. Its detoxification enzymes purify the blood and keep it free from substances that can cause cancer at various tissues sites within the body. As well, some 99 percent of any bacteria in the blood is intercepted and destroyed by the liver's Kupffer cells before the blood is allowed to recirculate.

In liver cells, and in other cells that fulfill detoxification duties, undesirable and harmful substances are neutralized by detoxification enzymes in a two-phase process. These enzymes are highly responsive to dietary and supplementation practices, which means we can actively counter their age-related decline. Phase I detoxification involves a group of enzymes called the mixed function oxidase enzymes, which comprise 50 to 100 different detoxifying enzymes. Essentially, these enzymes convert toxins either to less poisonous water-soluble forms, or to more active and dangerous metabolites such as free radicals, which are then neutralized in Phase II. Some Phase II detoxification enzymes act directly on other toxins—heavy metals, liver toxicants, bacterial and microbial compounds and endotoxins—converting them into compounds that the body can more easily eliminate. However, for the most part, Phase II is designed to intercept those harmful metabolites produced by Phase I, neutralize them, and prepare them for elimination through the urine or fecal matter.

Dietary factors and nutritional supplementation exert a profound influence on the ability of these systems to sustain performance and prevent the buildup of toxins and carcinogens in the bloodstream.

Among the foods known to promote Phase I detoxification enzymes are cabbage, cauliflower, turnips, kale, bok choy, broccoli, and Brussels sprouts. These cruciferous vegetables contain a substance called indole-3-carbinol, which stimulates detoxification to a significant degree. Studies show that individuals who consume higher amounts of these vegetables throughout their lifetimes have markedly less colon, breast, and prostate cancer incidence. Limonene, a flavonoid found in oranges and orange juice, also stimulates Phase I detoxification enzymes, as do niacin (vitamin B3), riboflavin (vitamin B2), and vitamin C. Interestingly, grapefruits and grapefruit juice, which contain a flavonoid called narangenin, slow Phase I detoxification by up to 30 percent.

To support Phase I and Phase II detoxification in the liver, follow these strategies:

- Take a daily high-potency multiple vitamin and mineral supplement that is enriched with a B-50 complex and antioxidants:
  - Vitamin C: 1,000 mg
  - Vitamin E: 400 I.U.
  - Selenium: 100-200 mcg
  - Molybdenum: 50-75 mcg
  - Beta-carotene: 10,000-20,000 I.U.

- After age 40, consider adding an immune-detox support supplement containing indole-3-carbinol (the active detoxifier in cruciferous vegetables) and milk thistle (standardized to 80 percent silymarin content).

- Drink a daily protein shake, rich in soy whey protein (provided you are not sensitive to these proteins). These proteins enhance liver function, strengthen the immune system, and reinforce the intestinal barrier to toxins. Soy isoflavones also assist the performance of many Phase II liver enzymes, making them more efficient.

Let's look at how supplementation with milk thistle and indole-3-carbinol can supercharge your body's detoxification capacity.

Milk Thistle

The medicinal use of milk thistle was acknowledged by the well-known seventeenth-century pharmacist, Nicholas Culpeper, who cited it as a useful agent for opening "obstructions" of the liver and spleen and for the treatment of jaundice. Even the Greeks and Romans noted its ability to protect against and repair certain liver conditions. More recently, scientific investigation of liver-related conditions in the 1960s led to the isolation of silymarin from the plant's ripe seeds. It is silymarin—a mixture of flavonolignans consisting chiefly of silibinin, silidianin, and silicristin—that improves liver health and boosts the detoxification capabilities of Phase II enzymes. To be effective, milk thistle extracts should contain a minimum of 80 percent silymarin content.

Here's why milk thistle is so important:

- **Antioxidant function:** Silymarin has been shown to be at least ten times more potent an antioxidant than vitamin E in the liver, stomach, and intestine. Experimental evidence has revealed that silymarin protects animals from liver damage after exposure to such diverse toxic chemicals as carbon tetrachloride, ethanol, galactosamine, and amanita phalloides and its toxins, a lethal agent found in toadstool mushrooms.

- **Liver glutathione:** Silymarin increases liver glutathione content by over 35 percent in healthy human subjects and by over 50 percent in rats. Glutathione is an active protein in both Phase I and Phase II detoxification processes and acts as an intracellular antioxidant that protects cells against dangerous free radicals from various sources. In many liver and immune-related diseases, glutathione liver concentrations are depleted, permitting faster disease progression. The ability of milk thistle to help restore glutathione levels makes it an effective treatment for various liver conditions.

- **Blocking leukotrienes:** Silymarin inhibits the formation of inflammatory chemicals called leukotrienes, thereby helping to control swelling and inflammation resulting from mechanical and chemical assaults.

- **Stimulating protein synthesis:** Silibinin stimulates the enzymes that cells use to replicate DNA and RNA, which in turn leads to new liver cell development. This means that the regenerative capacity of liver cells is enhanced with damaged cells repaired and old ones replaced.

- **Increasing superoxide dismutase concentrations:** Silymarin raises the concentrations of superoxide dismutase enzyme, a powerful intracellular antioxidant that neutralizes the superoxide anion—an aggressive and reactive free radical oxygen species. This action helps protect liver cells from the cumulative effects of free radicals as we age.

Milk thistle's influence on the liver is so powerful that it has been used therapeutically in the treatment of such serious ailments as cirrhosis and chronic and acute viral hepatitis, and cases in of sluggish liver or minor hepatic insufficiency—a term used by

European physicians and American naturopaths to describe a myriad of symptoms, including an ache beneath the ribs, fatigue, unhealthy skin appearance, general malaise, constipation, allergies, premenstrual syndrome, and chemical sensitivities. In addition, milk thistle has been beneficial in the treatment of psoriasis and other skin problems where toxins in the bloodstream trigger immune inflammatory reactions that aggravate these conditions.

I recommend daily milk thistle supplementation—300 mg per day, standardized to 80 percent silymarin content—to slow or prevent some of the major biological effects of aging and for its general health-promoting properties.

Indole-3-Carbinol

Indole-3-carbinol is a member of the class of naturally occurring sulfur-containing chemicals called glucosinolates. It is formed by the action of the myrosinase enzyme on the parent compound glucosinolates whenever cruciferous vegetables are crushed (for example, in chewing) or cooked. Indole-3-carbinol (and other glucosinolates) are antioxidants and potent stimulators of Phase I and Phase II detoxification enzymes in the liver and intestinal lining. It helps the body eliminate toxic compounds, including many carcinogens, and it acts as a phytoestrogen, reducing the ability of stronger estrogens to overstimulate reproductive tissues—the breast, cervix, uterus, and in males, the prostate gland. Observational and experimental studies indicate that it plays an important role in the prevention of reproductive organ cancers and colon cancer. Since breast, prostate, and colon cancer occur at higher rates in older populations, it is prudent to boost your body's defenses after age 40 by supplementing with 50 mg of indole-3-carbinol per day, in addition to the frequent consumption of cruciferous vegetables.

Immune and Nutrition Function

Like the body's detoxification system, the immune system also becomes less effective between the ages of 40 and 50, thanks to a decline in the function of the thymus gland and the cumulative effects of free radicals acting on our immune cells.

The thymus gland instructs certain immune cells to identify and kill germs that may enter the body and to identify and eliminate emerging cancer cells before they can pose a real threat. Furthermore, the thymus produces T-lymphocytes, a type of white blood cell that is responsible for fighting infections, in particular those from mold-like bacteria, yeasts (including Candidia Albicans), fungi, parasites, and viruses. It also secretes various hormones which have far-reaching positive effects on the entire immune system. Low levels of thymus gland hormones in the blood are associated with decreased immunity and increased susceptibility to infection.

Vitamin and Mineral Supplements

Researchers have established that the decline in thymus gland function can be modified to a significant degree by supplementing with the high-potency multivitamin and mineral recommended in Step 2. Supplementation with vitamin A, for example, prevents stress-induced premature shrinkage of the thymus and actually promotes its growth and regeneration. Studies examining zinc supplementation have discovered its many positive effects on immune function, including enhanced release of thymus hormones. Selenium supplementation is also known to stimulate white blood cell and thymus function. The National Health and Nutrition Examination Surveys have told us that a significant portion of the population do not ingest the recommended levels of these vitamins and minerals every day and few do so at levels are not sufficient to support high immune and thymus gland function.

In the 1980s and 1990s, a number of researchers explored the potential of specific vitamins, at supplemented levels, to improve immune system function and reduce the risk of infections and related diseases. They demonstrated that not only were certain vitamin deficiencies in animals associated with an increased incidence of disease, but that vitamin supplementation could reverse impaired immune system function in humans and animals. Vitamin E supplementation enhanced tissue immune system function in healthy older human subjects and rodents. Vitamin C supplementation significantly improved the respiratory condition of asthmatic patients. A combination of vitamins C and E increased blood levels of vital immune system agents (immunoglobulin G and complement 3) in healthy elderly women, enhanced the production of T-lymphocytes and white blood cells, and prevented the development of autoimmune disease in animals. And as we saw in Step 2, vitamin E supplementation reduces the production of the harmful prostaglandin hormone series-2, which tends to weaken the immune system, and it protects immune cells from free radical damage.

Several double-blind studies have shown that the elderly experience better immune function and a reduced rate of infection when taking a multiple vitamin and mineral formula. One study demonstrated that supplementation with 100 mcg of selenium and 20 mg of zinc, with or without additional vitamin C, vitamin E, and beta-carotene, led to fewer infections. Others reported improved outcomes when subjects were supplemented with either vitamin C, beta-carotene, vitamin A, lycopene, or vitamin B12.

The body of evidence suggests that all of these nutrients combined will provide the best possible benefits for immune function. This synergy was well illustrated by a study that was published in the *American Journal of Clinical Nutrition* in December 1996. Dr. Kee-Ching, G. Jeng and their colleagues recruited forty healthy male and female volunteers, aged 22 to 55 years, from the staff and students of the Taichung Veteran's General Hospital and Providence University in Taiwan. The subjects were administered either vitamin C (1,000 mg per day), or vitamin E (400 mg per day) alone, or vitamin C and vitamin E in combination at the dosages, for 28 days. Those receiving the combination of vitamin C and vitamin E had the most improved results in immune system function and demonstrated the lowest levels of free radical damage. This group also had the lowest production of prostaglandin E2. The conclusion of the researchers was that combined supplementation with vitamins C and E is more effective than supplementation with either vitamin alone in healthy adults. This finding is shared by other investigators, who have concur that nutrients work together to optimize the function of the immune system and improve overall health status.

Reishi Mushroom Extract

The Reishi mushroom (Ling Zhi or Ganoderma lucidum) has been used for thousands of years by herbal practitioners in China and Japan. It is listed as a "super herb" in China's pharmacopoeia because of its ability to modulate immune function and for its anti-cancer and liver-protective properties. Reishi mushrooms contain unique polysaccharides, carbohydrates which exert positive effects on the immune system. Other active constituents include the ganoderminc acids, classified as triterpenoids, which are compounds with a structure similar to steroid hormones.

Reishi mushroom extract boosts the cancer-cell-killing capacity of certain immune cells, increases their ability to identify and kill many microorganisms, and encourages the release of cytokines, hormones that act as signaling agents to improve immune system efficiency. Studies have revealed that reishi mushroom extract can reestablish normal white blood cell levels following radiation therapy, leading to its use as a cancer treatment by many practitioners in Asia.

To ensure that sufficient amounts of immune-strengthening agents are present you should use reishi mushroom supplements that are a standardized grade yielding at least 10 percent polysaccharide and four percent triterpene content.

Astragalus

The root of the astragalus membranaceous is a common herbal remedy in traditional Chinese medicine. Its key active ingredients include saponins, flavonoids, and polysaccharides. Astragalus can affect immune function in many ways: it enhances the ability of natural killer cells to destroy cancer cells and microorganisms; it encourages the proliferation of splenocytes, spleen cells that destroy foreign invaders; and it exhibits direct antiviral properties.

In human studies, astragalus supplementation has increased serum levels of various immunoglobulins, proteins that are an important part of our immune defense. IgM, IgE, and nasal secretions of IgA and IgG all contribute to immune function at various levels. When used as a daily preventive measure, astragalus has been shown to reduce the incidence of the common cold. It improves the responsiveness of lymphocytes in normal subjects and cancer patients, stimulates natural killer cell activity in normal subjects and those with lupus, and strengthens the immune system in individuals with AIDS and cancer. Like reishi mushroom extract, astragalus is safe to take on daily basis.

The combination of milk thistle, indole-3-carbinol, reishi mushroom extract and astragalus can boost immune function and detoxification and reverse certain aspects of age-related decline.

This is why I recommend that after the age of 40 you supplement your diet with a formula that fortifies these systems beyond the levels attainable by a high potency multi-vitamin and mineral alone.

Amount per two capsules:

- Milk thistle: 300 mg (standardized to 80 percent silymarin content)
- Indole-3-carbinol: 50 mg (standardized to 97 percent indole-3-carbinol content)
- Astragalus: 200 mg (2:1 extract)
- Reishi mushroom extract: 60 mg (standardized to 10 percent polysaccharide and four percent triterpene content)

3. Protecting the Prostate: Saw Palmetto, Pygeum Africanum, Beta Sitosterol, Soy Iso Flavones, Stinging Nettle, and a Healthy Lifestyle

The male prostate gland lies below the bladder and surrounds the urethra, that part of the male plumbing system that serves as a flexible pipe for the flow of urine out of the body. Enlargement of this walnut-shaped gland can put pressure on the urethra and obstruct the flow of urine as it exits the bladder, reducing the force of the urine stream and producing other symptoms (such as difficulty in initiating urination, or urgent urination). Enlargement of the prostate is an extremely common problem in men over the age of forty; it's due largely to age-related hormonal changes that occur in the male body. Many of the same age-related changes to the prostate gland that cause enlargement are also associated with the development and spread of prostate cancer.

Nearly 60 percent of North American men between the ages of 40 and 59 years will develop an enlarged prostate gland, also known as benign prostatic hyperplasia. By age 80, ninety percent experience significant symptoms. More alarming, 200,000 American men are diagnosed with prostate cancer every year and 30,000 die of it. Canadian statistics indicate that one in every eight men develops prostate cancer and one in 26 men in Canada die from this disease. Those who survive face formidable treatment choices, such as surgery or radiation which do not always work but which commonly case side effects, including impotence and incontinence. These numbers are expected to increase as the baby boom generation of North American men enters the prostate cancer risk years.

After age 40, blood levels of testosterone, the main male hormone, begin to fall. At the same time, blood levels of other hormones, such as estrogen, prolactin, luteinizing hormone, and follicle stimulating hormone, start to rise. These changes lead to greater concentrations of testosterone in the prostate gland and an increased conversion of testosterone to dihydrotestosterone (DHT) by the 5-alpha-reductase enzyme within prostate cells. The buildup of DHT stimulates the cells to divide and multiply at a faster rate than is considered normal or safe. More prostate cells mean not only prostate enlargement and its attendant problems, but more chances of cancerous DNA mutations. (When cells divide more quickly they make a greater number of genetic mistakes, with less time for DNA repair enzymes to correct them.) Indeed, males born with a genetic inability to synthesize DHT are immune to prostate cancer. DHT is also known to promote the spread of existing prostate cancer and the production of free radicals, a direct cause of cancerous mutations in the DNA of prostate cells.

The encouraging news is that attention to proper diet and the use of specific supplements can help block the conversion of testosterone to DHT and deliver other protective benefits to the prostate. There are several known natural agents that, when taken at the correct dosage and standardized grade, are proven effective in the treatment of enlarged prostate and have been associated with the prevention of prostate cancer or with its successful management.

Supplements that Block the Buildup of DHT

Saw Palmetto

Saw palmetto is a small palm tree with berries that contain various unsaturated fatty acids and sterols. Numerous studies have demonstrated that these fatty acids and sterols block the conversion of testosterone to DHT and exert other favourable influences on prostate health. Concentrated saw Palmetto extract is an established therapy for enlarged prostate conditions, and it has recently been used in trials with prostate cancer patients. A systematic review of saw palmetto and its effects was published in the *Journal of the American Medical Association* in the late 1990's. After evaluating studies from around the world, the authors concluded that saw palmetto produces improvements in urinary tract symptoms and urinary flow similar to those of the drug finesteride (also known as Proscar, prescribed for the treatment of enlarged prostate glands), with fewer adverse side effects. For example, erectile dysfunction rates are nearly five percent with finesteride use but approximately one percent with for saw palmetto. For the treatment of benign prostatic hyperplasia, the usual dose is 160 mg, twice daily, of saw palmetto extract (standardized to 90 percent fatty acids and sterols) or 320 mg, twice daily, of a standardized grade containing 45 percent fatty acids and sterols.

Pygeum Africanum

Pygeum africanum, a natural agent derived from the bark of the pygeum africanum tree, contains active compounds known as triterpenes, which have been demonstrated effective in the treatment of enlarged prostate in several human studies. The active ingredients in pygeum afri-canum reduce blood levels of leutinizing hormone and prolactin and suppress the synthesis of cholesterol in the prostate. Within the prostate the synthesis of cholesterol leads to a greater build of testosterone and DHT, as testosterone is made from cholesterol. By-products of cholesterol metabolism have also been shown to promote the degeneration of prostate cells, leading to prostate enlargement. Research has shown that pygeum africanum supplementation can reverse prostate enlargement problems. The usual dose for prevention and treatment is 100 to 200 mg per day (standardized to 12 to 14 percent triterpenes).

Beta-sitosterol

Beta-sitosterol is a common sterol that occurs naturally in saw palmetto, soy products, and other plant foods. Epidemiological and experimental studies suggest that it and other plant sterols offer protection against colon, prostate, and breast cancer. Recent findings published in the *Lancet* and the *British Journal of Urology* focused on its benefits for the prostate: when taken at a dosage of two mg three times a day, or 65 mg twice a day, beta-sitosterol reversed enlarged prostate symptoms. It does this by inhibiting the 5-alpha-reductase enzyme that converts testosterone to DHT and by blocking the formation of estrone hormone in fat cells, another mechanism that encourages the conversion of testosterone to DHT.

Soy Isoflavones

Soy products, including soy extract, contain several important isoflavones, among them genistein and diadzein. Genistein inhibits the accumulation of DHT and exhibits other properties that are related to the prevention of prostate disease and enlargement. Soy isoflavones are known to induce the programmed cell death of prostate cancer cells, while lowering testosterone and DHT stimulation, slowing the cell division rate of prostate cells and prostate cancer cells, and acting as an antioxidant.

Stinging Nettle

Stinging nettle (urtica dioica) is a natural agent that has been used successfully in European studies to reverse prostate enlargement. It is a weed whose aerial parts and roots contain its active ingredients, including specific flavonoids, sterols, lignans, fatty acids, polysaccharides, and lectins. Stinging nettle extract inhibits the ability of DHT to bind to the nuclei of prostate cells, thereby protecting their DNA material.

All-in-One Prostate Supplement

Men 40 years of age and older should take an all-in-one prostate supplement every day to counter the age-related changes that encourage the development of prostate enlargement and prostate cancer. A well-designed prostate support supplement will contain the following in a single capsule; I recommend two capsules per day:

- Saw palmetto – 320 mg (standardized to 45 percent fatty acids and sterols)
- Pygeum africanum – 100 mg (standardized to 14 percent triterpenes)
- Beta-sitosterol – 65 mg
- Soy extract – 100 mg (standardized to 10 percent isoflavone content)
- Stinging nettle extract – 30 mg (5:1 extract)
- Pumpkin seed extract – 25 mg
- Lycopene powder – 12.5 mg

This dosage is appropriate for the treatment of enlarged prostate conditions. For men with prostate cancer, four to six capsules per day may be used in conjunction with traditional medical treatment. Prostate cancer patients must check with their attending physicians before commencing a supplementation program of this kind.

Prostate Cancer

As we saw earlier, prostate cancer is the most frequently diagnosed cancer among men in Western countries, accounting for a third of all cancers that afflict them. In Africa, Eastern Europe, and Japan, the disease is far less prevalent, and research is showing us why.

In 1996, in an article in the *Journal of the National Cancer Institute*, Dr. W. Willet suggested that as many as 75 percent of prostate cancers could be prevented if men followed healthier nutritional practices. It appears that dietary and lifestyle factors influence not only the development of the disease but its rate of progression as well. Post-mortem studies have shown evidence of latent—that is, existing but not manifest—prostate cancer at similar levels in both high- and low-risk regions of the world. In other words, by their late forties, between 13 and 32 percent of all men will have cancer cells present in their prostate glands, regardless of where they live. (Some examples: in Singapore, this applies to roughly 13 percent of the male population; in Hong Kong, 16 percent; and in Sweden, 32 percent.) However, in low-risk areas, these latent cancer cells tend not to progress to a clinically significant malignant state, remaining dormant and non-life-threatening instead.

Another intriguing finding emerged from migration studies. In Japan, the incidence of serious prostate cancer is 80 percent lower than in North America. When men relocated from Japan to higher-risk Western countries and abandoned their traditional dietary habits, their incidence of prostate cancer approached that of North American men.

Diet, Lifestyle, and Prostate Cancer

A variety of nutritional and lifestyle factors have been strongly linked to the development of prostate cancer. To reduce the risk, be aware of the hazards to avoid and the habits to adopt.

- Alcohol: Data on alcohol consumption was collected by the Harvard Alumni Study, a project that followed 7612 Harvard alumni (mean 66.6 years) from 1998 through 1993. The results, published in 2001, revealed that men with moderate liquor consumption (between three drinks per week and three drinks per day) showed a 61 to 67 percent increased risk of developing prostate cancer compared to men who never or infrequently consumed alcohol. Wine and beer did not appear to be as dangerous as liquor, but men who consumed alcohol of any kind between 1977 and 1988 had a twofold increased risk of prostate cancer compared to those with almost no alcohol consumption.

- Heterocyclic amines: Animal studies confirm that heterocyclic amines from pan-fried meats are known carcinogens. In 2001, a study by Drs. K.T. Bogen and G.A. Keating provided evidence that higher intakes of heterocyclic amines among African-American males may partially explain why they experience prostate cancer at twice the rate of Caucasian males. U.S. blacks were shown to consume up to three times more heterocyclic amines from blackened meat and fish at ages less than 16 and over 30.

- Indole-3-Carbinol and Cruciferous Vegetables: In the journal Oncogene, Dr. SR Chinni and fellow researchers provided strong evidence to showed that the indole ring structures present in cruciferous vegetables may play an important role in the prevention of prostate cancer. Their study demonstrated that indole-3-carbinol can inhibit the growth of PC-3-type human prostate cancer cells by arresting their cell division cycle and hastening their demise through programmed cell death. They concluded that indole-3-carbinol could be an effective chemopreventive or therapeutic agent against prostate cancer—another incentive to consume cruciferous vegetables every day.

- Aerobic Fitness and Blood Pressure: A link between vascular disease and increased risk of prostate cancer has recently been reported suggesting that increased levels of excitation, which can lead to elevated blood pressure and heart rate, may overstimulate the testosterone and DHT activity of prostate cells as well. Heart rate and blood pressure may represent indirect markers of potentially harmful androgen activity in the prostate. Findings released in 2001 by the Cardiovascular Health Study of 2442 subjects demonstrated that men with a resting heart rate equal to or greater than 80 beats per minute had a 60 percent greater chance of developing prostate cancer during a 5.6-year follow-up period than those with a resting heart rate of less than 60 beats per minute. A moderate to high level of aerobic fitness appears to offer some protection against prostate cancer.

- Saturated fat: Numerous studies have linked a high-animal-fat diet to an increased risk of prostate cancer, most likely because higher intakes of saturated fat promote the overproduction of testosterone. Consuming only low-fat animal products, as outlined in the nutrition guidelines of this book, is the best course.

- Omega-3 fats: In contrast to the undesirable effects of saturated fat, omega-3 fats have been shown to inhibit the growth of prostate cancer in experimental studies. The results of one investigation published in the *Lancet* in June 2001, demonstrated that in a population of 6,000 Swedish men, those who regularly consumed fish (salmon, sardines, herring, mackerel, all rich in omega-3 fats) showed a 33 percent reduction in prostate cancer risk during the 30-year follow up period, compared to men who ate little or no fish.

- Soy intake and isoflavones: Higher intakes of soy products have consistently resulted in marked reductions in prostate cancer incidence. As reported in 2004 by CancerSci, a recent study that analyzed the dietary consumption of individual phytoestrogens by patients with and without prostate cancer pointed to the significant protective effect of the soy isoflavones genistein and diadzein, as well as the phytoestrogen coumestrol. Moreover, soy isoflavones may have a role as chemotherapeutic. In one case study, a 66-year-old prostate cancer patient took a phytoestrogen supplement (160 mg per day) for one week prior to radical prostatectomy surgery. There was evidence of a significant shrinkage of the tumour mass, suggesting tumour regression, when compared with the preoperative needle biopsy.

The traditional Asian diet contains an average isoflavone content of 50 mg per day. That dosage—obtained from soy-based foods, supplements containing soy extract, or soy protein shake mixes—is highly recommended as one means of prostate cancer prevention.

Prostate Antioxidants

Like other cancers, prostate cancer may arise when free radicals attack prostate cells, converting them into mutant cancer cells. The antioxidant lycopene, described in Step 2, is especially effective in protecting prostate cells from free radical damage. It concentrates in the prostate gland at levels much higher than those found in the bloodstream, making it a tissue-specific antioxidant in prostate health. Human studies such as the Physicians' Health Study and the Health Professionals' Follow-Up Study have shown a striking correlation between higher lycopene blood levels or intake levels (6.5 mg per day or more), and lower rates of prostate cancer development—as much as a 40 percent reduction. We know that tomatoes are an excellent source of lycopene; others include guava, papaya, red grapefruit, and watermelon. Remember that lycopene is a fat-soluble antioxidant (a sister compound to beta-carotene) and needs some fat in the stomach to be absorbed. When you eat these foods, make sure you consume a bit of allowable fat at the same time.

Soy isoflavones also provide antioxidant protection to the prostate gland, and two recent human intervention trials by Dr. L.C. Clark et al and Dr. O.P. Heinon et al respectively suggest that vitamin E supplementation (60 IU per day) and selenium supplementation (200 mcg per day) can reduce the risk of prostate cancer by 40 to 50 percent.

Other Prostate-Protective Nutrients

Zinc – The prostate gland contains a higher concentration of zinc than any other organ in the body. Zinc is required to maintain semen volume and testosterone synthesis. In some studies, men with prostate enlargement have shown lower levels of zinc. Its absence allows the 5-alpha-reductase enzyme to convert testosterone into DHT at increased rates. Moderate zinc supplementation can help reverse prostate enlargement; a total daily zinc intake of 25 to 30 mg a day is recommended for the management of the condition. A minimum of 15 mg a day from a high-potency multiple vitamin and mineral supplement is suggested for general prostate health.

Vitamin D – Epidemiological studies have revealed that where year-round sunlight intensity is low, the rate of prostate cancer is high. In North America, for example, the incidence of prostate cancer is much higher in regions above the fortieth degree latitude, which roughly divides the United States in half, north to south. This phenomenon, which exists for breast cancer and colon cancer as well, has been attributed to the influence of direct sunlight exposure on blood levels of vitamin D.

Experimental and animal research has demonstrated that in some types of prostate cancer the administration of vitamin D can transform malignant cancer cells to more normal prostate cells, inhibit prostate cancer cell replication, and suppress metastasis. Preliminary human studies have yielded encouraging results, but it is too soon to know if high-dose vitamin D supplementation (2,000 IU per day) is useful as an adjunct to prostate cancer treatment. As a means to help prevent prostate cancer, however, it is prudent to take a high-potency multiple vitamin and mineral each day that contains 400 IU of vitamin D. Each 400 IU elevates blood levels of vitamin D by 40 (nanomoles per litere, nmol/L . It is not uncommon to see low levels in the range of 15 to 45 nmol/L in individuals living in the northern United States and Canada. Cancer studies suggest that blood levels of vitamin D should be in the range of 85 to 110 nmol/L, which is also ideal for the prevention of osteoporosis. Men over the age of 40 who live in these high-risk regions of North America should consider taking an additional 400 to 600 IU of vitamin D every day, especially between October and May.

Lifestyle Decisions

Because of the prevalence of prostate gland enlargement and the almost certain growth in prostate cancer incidence, it is worth summarizing the preventative measures that can be taken. The following recommendations should be seriously considered by all men throughout their lifetimes:

- Follow a diet that is low in saturated fat.
- Remain at or near your ideal body weight.
- Drink alcohol in moderation or not at all.
- Consume tomato or tomato products on a daily basis, as well as other lycopene-containing fruits and vegetables.
- Use more soy products, such as tofu, veggie burgers, miso soup, soy nuts, and soymilk.

- After age 40, consider taking an all-in-one prostate support supplement that contains the herbal ingredients outlined in this chapter. It is vital that the herbal and accessory compounds be present in the correct dosages and standardized grades in order to be effective.

- Take a high-potency multivitamin and mineral that is enriched with the following antioxidants: vitamin E (400 IU), selenium (100 to 200 mcg), vitamin C (1000 mg), plus 15 mg of zinc and 400 IU of vitamin D.

- Eat cruciferous vegetables at least three times per week.

- Avoid pan-fried meats and other sources of heterocyclic amines (charred barbecued meats and blackened fish and meats).

- Stay fit, especially from a cardiovascular fitness standpoint, striving for a resting heart rate below 60 beats per minute.

4. Managing Menopause: Black Cohosh, Soy Isoflavones, and Gamma-Orzanol

Today men and women are enjoying greater longevity than ever, thanks to better sanitation and hygiene practices, advances in the fight against infectious diseases, modern medical care, and improved nutrition. Women can expect to live fully one-third of their lives after the onset of menopause, years that should be satisfying, productive, and blessed with a sense of wellbeing.

It can be a challenge to combat the age-related changes that occur at this stage of life, to cope safely with the uncomfortable physical symptoms of menopause, and to minimize the risk of osteoporosis, heart attack, breast cancer, and other health problems that are prevalent in women over 50. These changes result from the dramatic yet inevitable decline in the synthesis of estrogen, progesterone, and testosterone in the body. Adhering to a healthy diet and a regular exercise program while maintaining a positive mental attitude are important first steps, but these alone cannot deter or slow the profound effects of the aging process. Specific natural supplements should be added to the program when menopause arrives. To appreciate the difference supplements can make, it's useful to understand the physical alterations that occur in the body at the onset of menopause.

The Cause and Effects of Estrogen and Progesterone Decline

Throughout a woman's fertile years, the hypothalamus gland in her brain monitors her blood levels of estrogen and progesterone. At the end of every menstrual cycle, when it senses that these levels have dropped significantly, it releases hormones that prompt the pituitary gland to produce follicle stimulating hormone (FSH) and luteinizing hormone (LH). The release of FSH and LH into the bloodstream stimulates some of the immature egg cells in the ovaries to begin a maturation process that leads to one of the eggs outpacing the rest, bursting out of the ovaries around day fourteen and entering the fallopian tube. During this ovulation process, the egg secretes estrogen. If the egg is not fertilized by a sperm cell, it will eventually shrivel and die. When this occurs, estrogen levels in the bloodstream fall again, which the hypothalamus's cue to initiate another menstrual cycle by releasing the hormones that stimulate the release of FSH and LH from the pituitary gland.

Most of the estrogen in a woman's body is supplied by these developing and maturing egg cells, although small amounts are also secreted by the adrenal glands and fat tissue, sources that continue to make estrogen after the cessation of menstrual cycles. These amounts are minimal, however. During a woman's fertile years her daily estrogen secretion is 250 to 300 micrograms per day. After menopause, estrogen production—now from adrenal glands and fat tissue alone—drops to 20 micrograms per day, a 90 percent decline.

When a woman approaches the age of 50, her ovaries become less responsive to the influence of follicle stimulating hormone and luteinizing hormone. This means that even though there are about 10,000 immature egg cells remaining in her ovaries, they cannot be prompted to mature by FSH and LH. This lack of response by the immature egg cells at the outset of menopause simply sends the pituitary into overdrive, releasing greater amounts of FSH and LH, which contribute to the onset of hot flashes and other symptoms. Still, ovulation will not occur, and little or no estrogen will be secreted. The resulting drop in the body's estrogen levels has far-reaching effects on the acceleration of aging and the development of degenerative conditions, in addition to introducing a range of attendant ills (including reduced energy, forgetfulness, dry mucous membranes throughout the body, atrophy or thinning of the skin and vaginal tissue, decreased libido, changes in hair texture, mood swings, and anxiety). As if this weren't enough, the decline in estrogen also encourages the loss of calcium from bones, setting the stage for osteoporosis, and a decrease in the body's ability to clear cholesterol from the bloodstream, thereby raising the risk of heart attack and stroke.

What about progesterone? Where does it come from and what effects result from its decline during menopause? The part of the maturing egg follicle that is left behind in the ovary after ovulation occurs, known as the corpus luteum, is the primary source of progesterone in a woman's body. As with estrogen, when the egg cells become unresponsive to the effects of FSH and LH and stop maturing, there is a drop-off in progesterone secretion. At the onset of menopause, blood levels of progesterone fall from 1.6 nanograms per milliliter to 0.5 nanograms per milliliters, a decrease that further promotes the development of osteoporosis and is associated with reduced libido, and thinning skin.

Until recently, many in the medical profession encouraged the use of hormone replacement therapy to combat menopausal symptoms and the threat of osteoporosis in postmenopausal women. Although effective for these problems, hormone replacement therapy is now known to have inherent hazards that outweigh its benefits. The natural alternatives are all the more attractive when these dangers are examined closely.

The Dangers of Hormone Replacement Therapy

Women worldwide have recently had cause to reconsider hormone replacement therapy (HRT) as a means to reduce menopausal symptoms. Over the past decade, a growing number have turned to the use of herbal remedies as an alternative to HRT, and this interest in natural therapies is expected to rise in the wake of two alarming and widely reported studies. These studies confirmed previous suspicions that hormone replacement therapy increases the risk of breast cancer and that unopposed estrogen (that is, estrogen not given with progesterone, as is often the case for women who have undergone hysterectomies) substantially increases the risk of ovarian cancer.

In July 2002, researchers the National Institutes of Health announced that they were ending the long-term American Women's Health Initiative trial of 16,000 women who were taking hormone replacement therapy because they discovered, just over five years into the study, that there was a 26 percent increased incidence of breast cancer in the women using HRT compared to those receiving the placebo. Women taking HRT also showed a 41 percent increased incidence of stroke and a 29 percent increased incidence of heart attack (myocardial infarction), compared to women receiving the placebo.

Further alarming news about estrogen replacement therapy appeared in the July 17, 2002, issue of the *Journal of the American Medical Association*. In a follow-up study of 44,241 former participants in the Breast Cancer Detection Demonstration Project, researchers discovered that the use of estrogen replacement therapy (without the concurrent use of progesterone) increased the incidence of ovarian cancer. The longer the use of the therapy, the greater the risk of developing the cancer. This mirrored earlier findings from the Nurses' Health Study, which demonstrated that for every year a woman remained on HRT, her risk of developing breast cancer increased by 2.3 percent. Thus a postmenopausal woman taking HRT for 10 years had a 23 percent increased risk of developing breast cancer, compared to women who were non-users of HRT. After 20 years of HRT use, a woman's risk of developing breast cancer would be 46 percent greater than that of a woman who had never used HRT during her menopausal years.

Clearly there is a need for safe and credible alternatives to HRT to alleviate menopausal symptoms, to enhance a healthy appearance and an active sex life, and to help maintain high quality of life for as long as possible. ·Any nutrition, supplementation, or lifestyle recommendations designed to accomplish these objectives must first address the three major health concerns for women 50 years and older: breast cancer, osteoporosis, and heart disease.

Heart disease

In the premenopausal years, high blood estrogen levels increase the production of low-density lipoproteincholesterol receptors, which enable cells to extract harmful LDL cholesterol—known to increase the possibility of heart attack and stroke—from the bloodstream. In menopause, the drastic drop in estrogen levels appears to reduce the ability of cells to produce LDL cholesterol receptors, allowing cholesterol to accumulate in the bloodstream, stick to the walls of the arteries and cause a narrowing of the coronary blood vessels, which can lead to heart attack. In fact, heart disease is the number-one killer of postmenopausal women.

Since a high-saturated-fat diet is the main culprit in raising LDL cholesterol levels, postmenopausal women should adjust their diets to reduce saturated fat intake in order to keep their blood cholesterol levels below 200 mg per decilitre (5.2 milimoles per litre). Animal protein sources should be confined as much as possible to chicken, turkey, Cornish hen or fish, and all milk and yogurt products should be non-fat or 1% varieties. Avoid any cheese above three percent milk fat content, as well as butter, ice cream, whipping cream, regular chocolate products, items containing coconut or palm oil, and deep fried products of all types.

Increasing consumption of soluble dietary fiber can also reduce blood cholesterol levels by literally dragging cholesterol out of the body, as do bile acids which aid the synthesis of cholesterol in the liver. Soluble fiber is found in many fruits, especially apples, peaches, pears, and plums, and in vegetables, oat bran, psyllium husk fiber, ground flaxseeds, beans and peas. Remaining physically fit with regular aerobic exercise and staying at or near your ideal weight are equally important lifestyle factors in preventing heart attack and stroke in the postmenopausal years.

Osteoporosis

With one in four women affected by age 50, osteoporosis is reaching epidemic proportions in North America. Experts blame its widespread incidence on insufficient calcium intake and accumulation of bone early in life, especially between the ages of 11 and 24, and on the loss of calcium from bone during menopause. Canadian statistics indicate that complications arising from osteoporotic hip fractures, such as the development of pneumonia, claim more lives every year than breast and ovarian cancer combined. The lifestyle recipe to prevent osteoporosis in later life is this:

1. If you are not taking HRT, ingest a total of 1,500 mg of calcium a day from diet and supplements. Note that calcium carbonate and calcium citrate are absorbed equally well if taken with meals. Since calcium carbonate is less expensive, it represents a more economical source. However, if you have a previous history of kidney stones, calcium citrate may be preferred due to its greater solubility.

2. Supplement with 600 to 1,000 IU of vitamin D, necessary for the absorption of calcium from the intestinal tract. For general health reasons, take a high-potency multiple vitamin and mineral, which normally includes 400 IU of vitamin D. After menopause, top up that dosage with an additional 200 to 400 IU per day. Studies show that postmenopausal women ingesting these levels of vitamin D may reduce their risk of hip fractures by as much as 50 percent. A high-potency multiple vitamin and mineral (including extra antioxidant protection and a B-50 complex) contains other nutrients important to bone health, among them zinc, magnesium, and copper.

3. Perform weight-bearing or resistance exercises three to six times per week. Weight-bearing activities such as walking or jogging, and weight training exercises place increased stress on the spine and femurs, which respond by holding their calcium in the bone to help withstand the demand on their structures. Research suggests that postmenopausal women can increase their bone density without HRT by simply ingesting more calcium and performing a series of specific weight training exercises, twice a week. Focus on these five weight resistant stations at the gym: hip extension, knee extension, abdominal machine, back extension machine, and lateral pull down machine. Perform two sets of 10 repetitions at each station, at 80 percent of your maximal effort.

4. Supplement with a product that contains black cohosh and soy isoflavones. As we'll see shortly, the standardized grade of black cohosh and soy extract can reduce menopausal symptoms and also help to preserve bone mineral density.

Breast Cancer

Breast cancer incidence has increased by 40 percent in the United States in last 50 years, with one in every 403 women afflicted between ages 50 and 59, one in 266 women be-tween ages 60 and 69, and one in 220 at age 70 and over. Currently one in 9 women in North America is expected to develop breast cancer during her life-time, and one in 27 will die from the disease. It is the most frequently diagnosed cancer in women in this part of the world, accounting for 32 percent of all cancers in women.

It's well documented that women who are overweight during their postmenopausal years have roughly a three times higher risk of developing breast cancer. As fat mass increases, there is a greater conversion of the hormone androstenedione to estrone within fat tissue. Estrone hormone, one of three types of estrogens made by the female body, increases the cell division rate of breast cells. As we've seen, this means a greater chance of genetic mutations occurring. Once formed, estrone can be further converted into beta-estradiol, another powerful estrogen hormone that is associated with increased breast cancer risk. This is exactly the mechanism through which HRT was shown to raise the threat of breast cancer.

Consequently, postmenopausal women are advised to attain and maintain an ideal body weight and a body mass index below 25. The New York University Women's Health Study, one of the longest and most respected studies of its kind, suggested in a 1995 report that postmenopausal women with a body mass index higher than 24.87 had a three times greater risk of developing breast cancer within a five-year follow-up period than did postmenopausal women with a body mass index below 24.87. You can calculate your body mass index by dividing your weight (in kilograms) by your height (in meters) squared. For example, let us say your weight is 130 lbs, or 58.5 kilograms, and your height is 5'7", or 1.675 meters. The square of 1.675 is 2.8. Divide 58.5 by 2.8 to arrive at your body mass index of 20.89, well within the safe range.

Finally, avoiding the use of HRT is emerging as a significant factor in the prevention of breast cancer in postmenopausal women.

Safe and Effective Herbal Supplements for Menopausal Women

Although so far underutilized by medical doctors in the western world, the benefits of black cohosh, soy extract, and gamma-oryzanol are supported by substantial and convincing evidence from European and Asian studies. They have demonstrated an ability to significantly reduce menopausal symptoms, support bone density, lower high cholesterol, prevent atrophy and dryness of vaginal tissues, help maintain a radiant complexion, and improve overall vitality. Unlike HRT, these natural substances are not associated with an increased risk of breast cancer, ovarian cancer or heart disease.

Black Cohosh

Black cohosh is a plant that is found in northeastern North America; its thick fibrous stock has long been used for medicinal purposes by First Nations peoples, in particular the Cherokee and the Iroquois. The discovery of its value for gynecological complaints led to its use in the management of menopause, and North American phy-sicians prescribed black cohosh for this purpose in the early decades of the twentieth century. However, the proliferation of synthetic drugs and the rise in influence of pharmaceutical companies after the first and second world wars has created a medical education system in the U.S. and Canada that no longer pays credence to effective herbal remedies, among them black cohosh. Curiously, although black cohosh is native to North America, most of the clinical investigations of its efficacy have been performed in Germany, where it is the most widely used and thoroughly studied natural supplement for the management of these symptoms. Since 1956, over 1.5 million menopausal women in that country have used black cohosh extract with noted success and without significant side effects. Studies have pointed out that to be effective black cohosh must be standardized to contain 2.5 percent triterpene content. These triterpene compounds account for most of the herb's therapeutic and anti-aging effects.

Four major independent human studies in Germany have demonstrated the ability of black cohosh to help manage menopausal signs and symptoms. In the first (an open study where no placebo or other product was given to a control group), involving 131 doctors and 629 female patients, 80 percent of patients experienced improvement of the physical and psychological symptoms associated with menopause, within six to eight weeks of treatment with black cohosh extract. Significant reductions were reported in the frequency and intensity of hot flashes, profuse sweating, headache, vertigo, heart palpitations, tinnitus, nervousness and irritability, sleep disturbances, and depressive moods. Only seven percent of subjects reported mild transitory stomach complaints.

A second study, using a control group, compared the effects of black cohosh to estrogen replacement therapy (0.625 mg C.E.E.) [Conjugated equine estrogen]and diazepam (two mg) for 12 weeks. Black cohosh outperformed both Premarin (C.E.E.) and Valium (diazepam) using the Kupperman Menopausal Index, one of the standard assessment tools in clinical studies of menopause. (This quantitative assessment of menopausal symptoms measures a range of symptoms by grades of severity.)

The third study, this one double-blind, compared the effects of black cohosh to estrogen replacement therapy (0.625 mg C.E.E.) or a placebo over a 12-week period. In this study, black cohosh produced better results in controlling menopausal symptoms, as determined by the Kupperman Menopausal Index and Hamilton Anxiety Test, and produced greater improvement in the condition of the vaginal lining than estrogen or the placebo. In the black cohosh group, the number of hot flashes dropped from an average of five a day to less than one. In the estrogen group, the number fell from five to 3.5 hot flashes a day on average.

In the fourth study, also double-blind, black cohosh was compared to a placebo in a study following 110 women. Here again the black cohosh group demonstrated significant improvement in menopausal symptoms and blood hormone measurements. In addition to relieving hot flashes, it produced impressive age-reversal results on the vaginal lining as confirmed by vaginal smear analysis.

Black cohosh extract appears to mimic the effects of estriol, which is the weakest of the three forms of estrogen made by the body. The other two, estrone and estradiol, are powerful estrogens that can overstimulate breast cells and endometrial cells, encouraging cancer development. The triterpenes found in black cohosh act more like estriol, which does not overstimulate breast tissue and is not associated with an increased risk of breast and reproductive cancers.

Black cohosh extract also inhibits the oversecretion of luteinizing hormone (LH), proof of its estrogen-like properties. Remember that the pituitary gland secretes LH only when it senses that estrogen levels have significantly dropped. When a woman supplements with black cohosh extract, the hypothalamus and pituitary glands sense that estrogen activity is sufficient, and they respond by shutting down the over-secretion of LH. Remarkably, active constituents that are unique to black cohosh have also been shown to serve as building blocks for the synthesis of progesterone in the body. As there is a 66 percent decline in progesterone levels at menopause, black cohosh can help preserve progesterone balance, which is important to bone health, libido and psychological well-being.

Attempts have been made by certain interest groups to discredit black cohosh by questioning its safety. There is no doubt that the rising popularity of natural agents such as black cohosh and soy isoflavones is eroding the sales of HRT drugs and hurting the profitability of the companies who manufacture them. Medications to manage menopause represent huge revenues to the pharmaceutical industry, since they are prescribed for daily use for 30 years or more on average. That will add up to hundreds of millions of dollars as female baby boomers enter their late forties and fifties. To lure women back to pharmaceutical solutions to the problems of menopause—which, after the hormone replacement scare, has switched to the use of anti-depressant drugs, anti-anxiety drugs, and anti-bone resorption drugs—the companies are looking for any opportunity to discourage the use of soy and black cohosh. They have publicized the most trivial studies of questionable significance that call into question the safety of these natural substances.

Let's examine the real facts. Black cohosh has been recommended or prescribed in the United States for more than 100 years and was an official drug in the U.S. pharmacopoeia from 1820 to 1926, prior to the moves that allowed patented drugs, manufactured by pharmaceutical companies, to dominate the drug market. Over the years many studies have documented black cohosh's effectiveness and safety. Published reports from Germany have established its high safety profile and relatively few and infrequent side effects, which include nausea, vomiting, headaches, dizziness, and breast pain. No drug interactions are reported in the medical literature for black cohosh, adding to its record as a safe intervention for the management of menopausal symptoms, as well as for PMS, dysmenorrhea, and other female reproductive complaints.

Throughout its documented use by millions of women over the past 40 years, there has been no indication that supplementation with black cohosh increases the risk of breast cancer, any other female reproductive cancer, or heart disease and stroke. In fact, given the findings of the American Women's Health Initiative study, it has a safety profile superior to that of hormone replacement therapy. Additionally, all of the experimental studies performed to date involving the use of human breast cells and human breast cancer cells have shown that standardized extracts of black cohosh actually block the development of breast cancer or decrease the ability of breast cancer cells to divide and multiply.

Reporting in the journal *Breast Cancer Research and Treatment* in 2002, Drs. C. Bodinet and J. Freudenstein showed that black cohosh extract significantly inhibited the division and spread of human breast cancer cells. They also demonstrated that black cohosh enhanced the ability of the anti-cancer drug Tamoxifen to suppress the proliferation of breast cancer cells, while managing the hot flashes induced by Tamoxifen. These researchers concluded that black cohosh extract treatment may be a safe, natural remedy for menopausal symptoms in patients who have had breast cancer. Their experimental data suggested too that black cohosh should be considered as part of the treatment protocol when Tamoxifen is administered to patients who have had breast cancer in the past.

A study by Drs. D. Dixon-Shanies and N. Shaikh, published in 1999 in *Oncology Report*, also demonstrated that black cohosh extract blocks the growth of human breast cancer cells. They concluded that certain herbs, such as black cohosh extract and soy (particularly the genistein isoflavone), may have potential in the prevention of breast cancer. Based on such findings, some experts recommend that women use a well-designed black cohosh and soy isoflavone supplement as a preventive measure throughout their adult lives (unless contraindications are present) to discourage the development or spread of breast cancer. Theoretically, the anti-proliferative effects of these herbal agents acting on breast cells could give the immune system a better chance to destroy cancer cells before they have an opportunity to take hold and grow.

Another supporting study by Dr JE Burdette and colleagues demonstrated that the natural ingredients in black cohosh extract inhibit free radical damage to the DNA of human breast cells when exposed to menadione, a potent free radical source. These substances (methyl caffeate, caffeic acid, ferolic acid, cimiracemate A, fukinolic acid) exhibited powerful antioxidant effects, suggesting that black cohosh can protect against cellular mutations caused by reactive oxygen free radicals. Other studies examining the toxicity of black cohosh, using high dosages in rats over extended periods, concluded that black cohosh is nontoxic and safe for long-term use.

Overall, the body of evidence indicates that black cohosh is a safe and effective alternative to hormone replacement therapy as a natural anti-aging intervention for the management of menopausal symptoms and that it offers significant benefits when combined with other nutrients.

Soy Isoflavones

Soy extract is another natural alternative to hormone replacement therapy for the treatment of menopausal symptoms. In clinical trials, soy isoflavone products have been credited with reducing hot flashes by as much as 40 percent. Soy isoflavones also possess phytoestrogen (plant-based estrogen) characteristics. They act as a "selective estrogen receptor modulator" or SERM, stimulating beta estrogen receptors on reproductive and other tissues and helping provide weak estrogenic support to reproductive tissue and bones, without overstimulating breast and endometrial cells.

Among the additional benefits of soy isoflavones are an antioxidant protection against free radicals, the slowing of breast cell proliferation, a reduction of the synthesis of estrone hormone by inhibiting the estrogen synthase enzyme in fat tissue, and an increase in the detoxification of harmful chemicals and hormones. The historically low incidence of breast cancer among Asian women has been linked to the protective effects of soy products, a staple of the traditional Asian diet. Unfortunately, steep increases in breast cancer incidence and mortality have been reported more recently in urban areas of China, Japan, and Singapore, where women have increased their consumption of animal fat. Asian women living in North America, eating a North American diet, exhibit breast cancer rates as high as other North American women.

The same phenomena have been demonstrated by research into ovarian cancer incidence among Asian and North American women. A recent study by Drs X. Chen and J Anderson showed that the soy isoflavones genistein and diadzein independently reduced the proliferation of human ovarian cancer cells in vitro. Although ovarian cancer affects only about 2 percent of women in the U.S., it is the fourth-leading cause of cancer deaths among women, in part because it is so difficult to diagnose in its early stages. Indeed, more than 60 percent of ovarian cancers are not diagnosed until they reach an advanced and, too often, fatal stage. As many as 95 percent of cases are linked to nutrition and environmental causes, making the protective effect of soy isoflavones all the more important.

Finally, soy isoflavones support bone mineral density in postmenopausal women, and help keep cholesterol levels within a safer range.

Gamma-oryzanol

Gamma-oryzanol is derived from rice bran oil. In Japan, where much of the research on this natural agent has been done, it is an approved drug, routinely prescribed for the treatment of menopausal symptoms. In North America, it is classified as a natural health product.

Like black cohosh, gamma-oryzanol will reduce the secretion of luteinizing hormone by the pituitary gland and encourage endorphin release by the hypothalamus. Clinical trials reveal that 67 to 85 percent of women treated with gamma-oryzanol have experienced significant relief of menopausal symptoms; a bonus is that gamma-oryzanol supplementartion at the proper dosage can reduce high cholesterol levels by up to 12 percent. It too is an extremely safe and non-toxic natural agent that should be part of any formulation aimed at controlling menopausal complaints and improving the health status of women during the menopausal stage of life.

Daily Dosages of Menopausal Supplements

It is now possible to find combination supplement products that provide all three menopausal nutrients—black cohosh, soy isoflavones and gamma-oryzanol—in a single formulation. As these three nutrients work synergistically, a combination formula gives a woman the best possible chance of managing her symptoms and enhancing her wellbeing, without resorting to hormone replacement therapy. Not all individuals respond equally to natural supplementation; however, in my experience, the majority of women report extremely positive results with the following dosages and standardized grades in a single all-in-one capsule. Menopausal and postmenopausal women should take two capsules per day.

- Black cohosh extract: 80 mg (standardized to 2.5 percent triterpene content)

- Soy extract: 250 mg (yielding 25 mg of soy isoflavones)
- Gamma-oryzanol: 150 mg

This combination of nutrients can be used safely as a viable alternative to HRT and by women who have contraindications to estrogen replacement therapy (those suffering fibrocystic breast disease, endometriosis, uterine fibroids, liver or gallbladder disease, pancreatitis, or unexplained uterine bleeding). Monitoring of bone density and blood lipids should be performed periodically. As well, women taking HRT may want to use this formula for general nutrient support, in order to acquire important isoflavones and related phytoestrogens to protect their breast tissues from the proliferative effects of HRT.

The only precautionary note is that this supplement cocktail should not be taken by women who have been afflicted with breast cancer or ovarian cancer, unless approved by their oncologist. It may be safe for breast and ovarian cancer survivors, and some research argues that it may in fact help reduce the risk of recurrence of breast cancer. However, until further study results are available, we cannot be certain that the use of this supplement combination is appropriate for breast cancer and ovarian cancer survivors.

To summarize, this supplement formula is highly recommended:

- as a natural alternative to estrogen replacement or HRT for postmenopausal women who demonstrate normal bone density or osteopenia (minimal or marginal bone loss);
- as an important source of phytoestrogens and phytonutrients for women of all ages to help reduce the risk of female-related diseases (cut the dosage in half for women 15 to 49 years of age);
- as a supplement for women with PMS, fibroids, endometriosis and fibrocystic breast disease;

- as an alternative treatment for postmenopausal women with contraindications to estrogen replacement therapy;
- as a dietary adjunct to estrogen replacement therapy or the birth control pill, to help tone down the over-stimulation effect of these drugs on breast and uterine tissues.

Unsafe Herbs for Menopause

There are other herbal agents in the marketplace that can help manage women's health problems, including meno-pausal symptoms, but virtually all are associated with significant and sometimes dangerous side effects or drug-nutrient interactions. Avoid red clover isoflavones and angelica species (dong quai), both of which have potent anti-coagulent effects and can increase the risk of bleeding disorders. These herbs taken on their own or in conjunction with other anti-coagulant drugs, such as aspirin, put women at risk of internal bleeding. The presence of coumarins in these herbs also adds to the possibility of severe sun-induced dermatitis (skin rash). Licorice root frequently causes high blood pressure after prolonged use.

Final Considerations

At or before age 50, women should have a bone mineral density test to determine their bone status. If osteoporosis is not found, then most women can simply follow the lifestyle program outlined in this section as part of their anti-aging and prevention program. In instances where significant bone loss has already occurred, the attending physician may wish to consider the use of biphosphonate drugs which can slow future calcium loss, or Raloxifen or other SERMs (such as Tamoxifen). All postmenopausal women should have their bone density tracked periodically to monitor the effectiveness of the program to which they are subscribing, whether it includes natural substances or conventional drugs. Blood work to determine fasting cholesterol and triglyceride levels and other biomarkers of cardiovascular disease should part of that regular screening.

5. Vitamin D for the Prevention of Osteoporosis and Cancer

Frequently underestimated and underappreciated, vitamin D acts as both a vitamin and a hormone. It plays a strong supporting role to calcium in the maintenance of bone density and deterring the processes that can lead to the development of various cancers. There is evidence to suggest that high vitamin D blood levels can also reduce the risk of multiple sclerosis, thanks to its positive effects on immune system function.

Until your mid-forties, the amount of vitamin D contained in a high-potency multivitamin and mineral, plus that derived from dietary sources (such as fortified dairy products and fish), is usually sufficient to maintain healthy bones and help discourage the establishment of cancer cells. After age 45, however, the alpha-hydroxylase enzyme in the kidneys that converts vitamin D to its most active form—1,25 dihydroxy vitamin D, also known as calcitriol—becomes less active. The resulting decline in the synthesis of calcitriol in the kidneys is a major contributor to the development of osteoporosis in women and men after 50 and to the risk of cancer in later life. It's possible to compensate for the age-related drop in calcitriol synthesis by raising levels of a less potent form of the vitamin, known as 25-hydroxy vitamin D, but consuming adequate amounts of vitamin D should be a lifelong concern.

Vitamin D deficiency has been described as an unrecognized epidemic in adult women of childbearing years (15 to 49) in the U.S., and researchers suspect it is equally prevalent among males of the same age. Older individuals are at risk due to vitamin D deficient diets, reduced sunlight exposure, and the decline in the conversion of vitamin D to calcitriol with age. Furthermore, many drugs inhibit the action or absorption of vitamin D. It is well known that cortisone or prednisone therapy interferes with the metabolism of vitamin D, as do barbiturates and anticonvulsants. All cause an increased breakdown of vitamin D and its metabolites and so increase osteoporosis risk. Other drugs that reduce vitamin D's effectiveness:

- Allopurinol
- Bile acid sequestrants (e.g., Cholestyramine and colestipol)
- Cimetidine and other H-2 antagonists
- Oral contraceptives
- Heparin
- Hydroxychloroquine
- Indapamide
- Isoniazid
- Mineral oil
- Neomycin
- Thiazide Diuretics
- Rifampin– (may reduce blood vitamin D levels by 70 percent)
- Orlistat– (reduces blood levels of vitamin D)

Several surveys have shown that a large percentage of adults of all ages have inadequate vitamin D in their blood to prevent osteoporosis, as well as prostate, breast and colon cancers. Research conducted at Boston's Massachusetts General Hospital found that 57 percent of people hospitalized for a variety of reasons were vitamin D deficient. Of those, 37 percent had consumed the recommended daily amounts of vitamin D (200 IU per day for adults under the age of 50, 400 IU per day for adults 51 to 70, and 600 IU for adults over 70). These levels are too low to guard against vitamin deficiency and osteoporosis and certainly insufficient to reduce the risk of cancer.

Vitamin D and Bones

Vitamin D's most familiar function is to aid in the absorption of calcium for bone development and density. One of its traditional sources, cod liver oil, has been used since the Middle Ages as a safeguard against rickets, a disease of infancy and childhood that we now know is caused by vitamin D deficiency. When fibrous bone or cartilage goes without sufficient calcium and other minerals, it fails to form hard, mature bone. The pull of muscles and the simple weight of gravity will bend and distort the bones as the child grows. In 1930, vitamin D was isolated and identified as the fat-soluble compound that made cod liver oil an effective protection and treatment for the disease.

However, it's not just infants and young children who need vitamin D. It's essential at every stage of life, to increase bone mineral density to its maximum at around age 24, to maintain it through the young adult years, and to prevent the loss of calcium from the bones after age 50. Your lifetime vitamin D status is critical to the integrity of your bones and other hard tissues. Here's how it works:

- Vitamin D in the bloodstream assists the absorption of calcium and phosphorous by stimulating the synthesis of calcium-binding protein in intestinal cells. Insufficient vitamin D blood levels can set the stage for the development of osteoporosis and related bone fractures.

- Vitamin D regulates the metabolism of calcium and phosphorous, both vital for neuromuscular function and mineralization of bone, nails, and teeth.

- Vitamin D acts directly on bone, aiding in its formation and repair. When necessary, it will trigger the release of calcium from bone to help maintain blood calcium levels within the normal range, a function it shares with parathyroid hormone.

Let's look at some recent research that underscores these benefits. In 1994 Dr. M. Chapuay and fellow research-ers reported the results of a study of 3,720 elderly women living in nursing homes. Those who received 1,200 mg of calcium plus 800 IU of vitamin D each day experienced a 43 percent reduction in hip fractures over a three-year period compared to those not taking these supplements. Another study, conducted by Dr. B. Dawson-Hughes et al and published in 1995, demonstrated that supplementation of postmenopausal women with 700 IU of vitamin D daily reduced the annual rate of hip fractures from 1.3 percent to 0.5 percent, a difference of nearly 60 percent. Another Dawson-Hughes investigation combined the daily supplementation of 500 mg of calcium with 700 IU of vitamin D and revealed a significantly reduced hip fracture rate in men and women taking the combination compared to the placebo group at the end of a three-year follow-up period.

After the age of 45 it is extremely important for both men and women to increase their vitamin D supplementation. You will recall the alarming statistic that osteoporosis affects one in four women over the age of 50 and one in eight men over the age of 50. However, the benefits of increased vitamin D supplementation don't end with the prevention of osteoporosis.

Vitamin D and Cancer

Vitamin D receptors exist on intestinal cells, as we've learned, and they are also present in other tissues and organs, including the brain, pancreas, skin, gonads, prostate, stomach, colon, breast, kidney, connective tissue, parathyroid gland, mononuclear cells, and activated T and B lymphocytes. Recent studies indicate that these tissues are able to convert 25-hydroxy vitamin D, extracted from the bloodstream, into calcitriol for their own needs. Calcitriol exerts a number of anti-cancer effects on local tissues: it slows the rate of replication of the tissue's cells, an effect associated with decreased cancer development; it has been shown to slow the rate of replication of human prostate, breast and colon cancer cells under experimental conditions; and it promotes newly formed cells to mature to their full adult potential, which also decreases the chance of these cells being transformed into cancer cells by some external influence. Calcitriol also favourably affects immune function, which is thought to account for some of its anti-cancer properties, including its ability to transform the appearance of human prostate cancer cells back to healthy, non-malignant-looking cells and to inhibit their replication in experimental studies, an effect that is lost once the calcitriol is no longer administered.

Some of the earliest research linking optimal vitamin D status with protection against cancer was conducted by Drs. C.F. and F.C. Garland. F.C. Garland was among the first to examine the effects of geographical location on cancer incidence, tying sun exposure and resulting vitamin D synthesis to cancer prevention. Together, the Garlands have undertaken several studies of vitamin D and cancer, among them one described in 1999 in the Annals of the New York Academy of Sciences. It showed that daily intake levels of 800 IU of vitamin D plus 1,000 to 1,200 mg of calcium prevents the development of colon cancer, and that 800 IU a day of vitamin D is the intake level that is associated with a significant decrease in the incidence of breast and prostate cancer, as well as enhanced survival rates for breast cancer.

The evidence that vitamin D reduces the incidence of colon cancer has been strengthened by the findings of several large human studies. Dr. C.F. Garland's Chicago-based Western Electric Study followed 1,954 men over a 19-year period, examining various risk factors for colon and rectal cancers. This study revealed that dietary vitamin D and calcium were independent factors in assessing colon cancer risk. Subjects who ingested more than 3.75 mcg (150 IU) of vitamin D per day from dietary sources experienced a 50 percent reduction in the incidence of colon cancer, compared to men ingesting less. A daily intake of 1200 mg of calcium was associated with a 75 percent reduction in colon cancer incidence. In his Washington County Maryland Study, which tracked 25,620 volunteers from 1975 to 1983, Dr. Garland reported that the risk of colon cancer was reduced by 75 percent in men and women who had blood levels of vitamin D between 67.5 and 80.0 nmol/L, and by 80 percent in those with blood levels of vitamin D between 82.5 and 102.5 nmol/L.

An Italian study by Dr. C. La Vecchia published in 1997 in *The International Journal of Cancer* compared the dietary habits of 2,053 colon and rectal cancer patients with 4,154 individuals who were free from colon cancer but who lived in the same vicinity and were admitted to the same hospital with other health issues. The results showed that high intakes of antioxidants (carotenes and vitamin C) as well as calcium and vitamin D were associated with a 54 percent reduction in colon cancer incidence.

A 2000 review of the Nurses' Health Study by Dr. E.A. Platz confirmed that women with low blood levels of vitamin D had a significantly higher incidence of colon cancer. This came to light when women who had provided blood samples in 1989 and 1990 later underwent endoscopic exams between 1989 and 1996.

Most recently, a 2003 paper in the *Journal of the American Medical Association* reported on the results of a study of 3,121 patients, aged 50 to 75 years, who were tested at thirteen Veterans Affairs medical centers across the United States between 1994 and 1997. The subjects showed no symptoms of colon cancer, but colonoscopy examination revealed that 329 participants had advanced cases of the disease. Those with a close family history of colon cancer or who smoked and drank alcohol at moderate to high levels were all at high risk of developing it. Those who ate more than 4.2 grams of cereal fiber every day or who were frequent users of non-steroidal anti-inflammatory drugs such as aspirin demonstrated significantly lower rates of colon cancer development, as did those who ingested more than 645 IU of vitamin D from food and supplements on a daily basis. Higher intakes of calcium were also shown to be protective, but to a lesser degree in this study.

Reviewing the extensive scientific evidence pertaining to vitamin D and cancer in the July 2002 edition of the *American Journal of Clinical Nutrition*, Dr Michael Holick of Boston University Medical Center stated that the production of calcitriol may be essential for the regulation of cellular health, thereby decreasing the risk of developing cancers. Though it's not widely acknowledged by health professionals or generally known by members of the public, high intakes of vitamin D and optimal blood levels of 25-hydroxy vitamin D have demonstrated a strong influence on the prevention of breast, colon, and prostate cancer, as well as osteoporosis.

The data is accumulating to show that vitamin D is also important in the prevention of ovarian cancer and multiple sclerosis. For example, in a study released in 2004, Dr K.L. Munger and colleagues showed that participants in the Nurses' Health Study who ingested 400 IU of vitamin D from supplements each day (from a multivitamin product) showed a 40 percent reduction in risk of multiple sclerosis compared to women who did not use supplements containing vitamin D. Other human and animal investigations have confirmed the effects of vitamin D on immune function that are consistent with preventing multiple sclerosis.

The Sources of Vitamin D

Moderate exposure to sunlight is the most natural way to restock your vitamin D stores; indeed, research has shown that vitamin D from sun exposure is the most potent in terms of preventing internal cancers as well as osteoporosis. Evolutionary theory suggests that as our dark-pigmented African ancestors migrated farther from the equator, those who possessed the genetic mutation for lighter skin were the ones who survived: the weaker sunlight could penetrate their skin more easily and vitamin D synthesis could occur. Today, for example, Scandinavians sport the fair skin that allows them to live in a region where sunlight intensity is relatively feeble.

To achieve the greatest possible vitamin D synthesis in the skin, simply enjoy 15 to 20 minutes of direct sunlight exposure on your face, arms and legs, three times a week. (This degree of exposure is not typically associated with an appreciable risk of skin cancer.) Unfortunately, few of us can hope for this amount of sunshine, especially those who live above the fortieth parallel where sunlight intensity between October and May is inadequate to make vitamin D in the skin. We have to look to other sources.

Among the preferred dietary sources are fish, vitamin D-fortified dairy products, and supplements. Fatty fish such as salmon and mackerel are rich in vitamin D and may be eaten three to four times a week to help meet the body's requirements. Fortified milk, despite its claims to contain 100 IU in every eight ounces, has been found to vary widely in vitamin D content depending on season, the breed of cow, the animal's diet, its exposure to sunlight, and the procedures used in fortification. The most reliable source of consistent and essential vitamin D levels is a supplement.

Low-Fat Food Sources of Vitamin D

Foods	Approximate I.U. of Vitamin D per 3.5 oz.
Sardines (canned)	1150-1570
Mackerel (raw)	1100
Salmon (fresh)	154-550
Salmon (canned)	220-440
Herring (fresh)	315
Herring (canned)	330
Shrimp	150
Halibut	44
Chicken	50-67
Oysters	5 IU per 3-4 medium sized oysters
Non-fat and 1% milk	up to 100 IU per ounces and yogurt (Vitamin D fortified)
Low-fat cheese (less than 4% 12-15 milk fat)	

Ensure Optimal Vitamin D Status by Supplementing after Age 45

Establish your vitamin D status with an annual blood test to measure circulating levels of 25-hydroxy vitamin D. Abundant research shows that adults who maintain levels in the range of 85 to 120 nmol/L have a significantly lower risk of developing osteoporosis, breast cancer, ovarian cancer, prostate cancer, colon cancer, and multiple sclerosis.

To ensure that your blood levels are within this protective range, it is important to increase your vitamin D supplementation to 800 to 1,000 IU per day after the age of 45. To the 400 IU of vitamin D from a high-potency multiple vitamin and mineral, add another daily supplement that contains 400 to 600 IU in a formulation that also provides an extra 500 to 700 mg of calcium. If the product contains additional magnesium, zinc and other bone support nutrients, so much the better.

Dr. Michael Holick points out that vitamin D consumption is completely safe up to 2,000 IU a day for ages one year and above, and that the risk of vitamin D toxicity has been greatly exaggerated by many health policy makers. Vitamin D toxicity has never occurred at blood levels below 250 nmol/L, so there is a wide margin of safety should you choose to implement vitamin D supplementation at 1,000 IU per day as recommended.

Personally, I derive 500 mg of calcium and 400 IU of vitamin D every day from a high-potency multiple vitamin and mineral supplement. Since I am older than 45 and my body no longer efficiently converts 25-hydroxy vitamin D to 1,25 hydroxyvitamin D, I take two caplets of an additional supplement that contains the following nutrients. In each caplet:

- 200 IU vitamin D
- 250 mg calcium
- 100 mg magnesium
- 2.5 mg zinc

6. Glucosamine Sulfate for Joints and Blood Vessels

Another age-related condition that is engineered into our genetic program is osteoarthritis. Also known as degenerative arthritis, osteoarthritis is the most common joint disease in humans and vertebrate animals. Its symptoms become increasingly prevalent after 45 and nearly half the population will suffer from it by age 65. Virtually everyone who lives past the age of 75 will develop it to some degree. Because of its prevalence, let's begin by examining the causes and remedies for this condition.

Glucosamine Sulfate and Osteoarthritis

In the past the development of osteoarthritis has been accepted as simple wear and tear on the joints of the body, but recent evidence suggests that it is caused by complex changes in the repair mechanisms that keep joints functioning smoothly. With age there comes a decline in the ability of cartilage cells in the joints to manufacture sufficient amounts of a substance called glucosamine sulfate. Under normal conditions, our cartilage cells continually synthesize glucosamine sulfate, one of the raw materials needed to make chondroitin sulfate, an important component of cartilage. The cartilage in our joints consists mostly of a tough protein material called collagen, which provides the structural backbone of joint cartilage. Chondroitin sulfate fills in the space between the collagen fibers, just as mortar fills in the spaces between the bricks of a house, and it increases the joint's shock-absorbing capabilities. Because old collagen fibers and old chondroitin sulfate are continually broken down by the body, we need to support the systems that manufacture both throughout our lifetimes.

By age 40 the rate of glucosamine sulfate synthesis is slowing and the production of chondroitin sulfate is much reduced. The soft, rubbery, shock-absorbing joint cartilage at the ends of our bones becomes thinner and gradually erodes, reducing the normal joint space between bones and allowing them rub against each other, causing pain and inflammation. Erosion of the joint cartilage also leads to the joints becoming tight, less flexible, even disfigured, with accompanying morning stiffness and loss of normal range of motion. Osteoarthritis doesn't mean just chronic pain and suffering, but a much reduced quality of life, restricting an individual's ability to perform work-related tasks or enjoy any number of recreational activities.

Many studies have demonstrated that glucosamine sulfate supplementation can compensate for the impaired glucosamine synthesis that occurs after age 40, providing cartilage cells with the ability to make more optimal levels of chondroitin sulfate and thereby slow or reverse the aging effects on our joints that lead to osteoarthritis. In fact, research suggests that glucosamine sulfate is an effective natural treatment for individuals who already suffer from osteoarthritis and joint cartilage injuries.

Glucosamine is a small and simple molecule that is readily absorbed from the gastrointestinal tract: it's been demonstrated that 90 to 98 percent of glucosamine sulfate is taken up intact. (By contrast, less than 13 percent of chondroitin sulfate is absorbed from the intestinal tract, making it significantly less effective than glucosamine sulfate as an agent in the prevention and management of osteoarthritis.) Once absorbed, glucosamine circulates through the bloodstream, where it can be taken up by the cartilage cells and contribute to the production of chondroitin sulfate. In addition, glucosamine sulfate is required for the synthesis of hyaluronic acid by the synovial membrane of the joint. Hyaluronic acid increases the viscosity of the synovial fluid and thus reduces the stress on the cartilage and related joint structures.

Investigations on the efficacy of glucosamine have used it in the form of glucosamine sulfate, a manufactured compound of glucosamine and the mineral sulpher. Only glucosamine sulfate is approved as a treatment for osteoarthritis in more than 70 countries around the world, where it has been used by millions of people for more than 20 years. Glucosamine sulfate delivers glucosamine to the joint cartilage, along with the mineral sulfur, a nutrient that stabilizes the connective tissue matrix of cartilage, tendons, and ligaments. The popularity of sulfur hot springs and the recent demand for methlyl sulfonyl methane (MSM) among arthritis patients offer strong anecdotal evidence that sulfur can help alleviate arthritis symptoms to a significant degree; indeed, preliminary trials with oral MSM in humans appear to support these endorsements. Other forms of glucosamine such as N-acetyl-glucosamine and glucosamine hydrochloride are available, but at present there is insufficient evidence to support their use and neither provides the benefits of sulfur.

Glucosamine sulfate has been the subject of more than 300 scientific investigations and over 20 double-blind clinical studies. In a comprehensive analysis of glucosamine clinical trials in the treatment of osteoarthritis published in the *Journal of the American Medical Association* in 2000, Dr. T.E. McAlindon and colleagues indicated that glucosamine sulphate supplementation reduced the symptoms and signs of osteoarthritis by 40.2 percent on average, compared with a placebo.

Glucosamine sulfate supplementation has also been investigated in head-to-head studies against non-steroidal anti-inflammatory drugs (NSAIDs) such as aspirin and ibuprofen for the treatment of osteoarthritis. In a number of these trials, glucosamine sulphate produced better results in relieving pain and inflammation, without the adverse side effects that are frequently encountered with NSAIDs such as gastritis, peptic ulcer, bleeding and erosion of the intestinal lining, liver and kidney toxicity, and tinnitus. In a 1998 therapeutic investigation conducted by Dr. G.X. Qiu and others involving 178 Chinese patients suffering from osteoarthritis of the knee, a group given a daily dose of 1,500 mg of glucosamine sulfate experienced greater relief of their symptoms than did another group given ibuprofen at 1,200 mg per day. In this study, glucosamine sulfate was also better tolerated than ibuprofen: sixteen percent of the ibuprofen group dropped out due to adverse side effects from the drug, while six percent of the glucosamine group withdrew. The authors concluded that glucosamine sulfate is a selective intervention for osteoarthritis, as effective for the symptoms of the disease as NSAIDs but significantly better tolerated. Glucosamine sulfate therefore seems particularly suited for the long-term treatment needed in osteoarthritis.

In answer to the skepticism of some in the medical profession who questioned the validity of the initial glucosamine research conducted in Europe and Asia, Dr. J.Y. Reginster and fellow researchers at the World Health Organization's Collaborating Center for Public Health Aspect of Osteoarticular Disorders in Liege, Belgium, published their findings in the journals *Arthritis and Rheumatology* and *Lancet* in 1999 and 2001 respectively. Their three-year study was a large, randomized-control intervention trial analysis of 212 patients with knee osteoarthritis. It was placebo-controlled, double-blind, and prospective in nature. Weight-bearing and antero-posterior radiographs of each knee were done at one and three years; joint space width was measured. Symptoms and functional status were scored every four months using the Western Ontario and McMaster University Osteoarthritis index. The two groups—a glucosamine sulphate group and a placebo group—began with comparable baseline conditions, but after three years the glucosamine group showed no further joint space narrowing. The placebo group exhibited increased joint space narrowing and evidence of disease progression. As well, symptoms worsened in the placebo group while the glucosamine group experienced a marked reduction in symptoms over the three-year period, with no untoward side effects. This was a landmark study that finally convinced the medical community that glucosamine sulfate was an effective natural agent for the treatment of osteoarthritis.

Glucosamine Sulphate, Blood Vessels, and Other Health Benefits

The clinical use of glucosamine supplementation may extend beyond its application as an effective intervention to halt joint cartilage destruction and help regenerate new cartilage in osteoarthritis cases. Glucosamine sulfate is required for the synthesis of other substances that are integral components of the filler material between skin cells in the epidermis and collagen and elastin fibers in the dermal layers of the skin. Glucosamine is also part of the matrix material that supports the intestinal tract lining and the walls of blood vessels; experimental studies and human anecdotal evidence support its application for post-surgical wound healing.

There is also experimental and anecdotal evidence to suggest that glucosamine sulfate supplementation may be beneficial as part of a nutritional regime for the management of inflammatory bowel diseases. It's been suggested that glucosamine supplementation can strengthen the basement membrane of gut blood vessels, helping prevent the leakage of blood into the intestinal tract and inflammatory immune reactions. Further, glucosamine has been shown to have a healing effect on the lining of the intestinal tract itself: anecdotal evidence supports the trial of glucosamine in both Crohn's disease and ulcerative colitis.

Finally, glucosamine sulfate supplementation may reduce the chances of blood vessel fragility, associated with the stroke and vein disorders that frequently occur with advancing age.

Side Effects, Toxicity, and Contraindications to the Use of Glucosamine

The reported adverse side effects from the use of glucosamine sulphate are generally mild and infrequent. These include minor gastrointestinal upset, drowsiness, skin reactions, and headache. Glucosamine sulfate is nontoxic at prescribed doses and safe for patients allergic or sensitive to sulfa drugs or sulfate-containing food additives. The word sulfate in this instance indicates the presence of the mineral sulfur, not the sulfa compounds used in sulfa drugs or sulfate-containing food additives. All body cells contain the mineral sulfur and consequently it's not possible to be allergic to it.

However, glucosamine sulfate is manufactured from the chitin exoskeleton of shellfish, such as lobster, crab, and shrimp. A person with severe allergies to shellfish may be sensitive, although the pharmaceutical grade of glucosamine is generally devoid of shellfish contaminants. Nevertheless, caution should be exercised in these cases.

A few preliminary animal experiments and human trials on healthy individuals reveal that glucosamine supplementation may increase insulin resistance in some individuals by down-regulating the synthesis of insulin receptors. In large clinical trials, this has not surfaced as a concern and no indication of pronounced glucose intolerance has been demonstrated in the many well-documented glucosamine studies, including the Reginster study and the comprehensive analysis published by the *Journal of the American Medical Association*. Some doctors have advised their patients not to take glucosamine if they are diabetic, but this is an unwarranted caution since many diabetic patients have benefited from the use of glucosamine without any adverse effects on their blood sugar. In fact, if glucosamine can relieve the pain and disability of osteoarthritis that is preventing a diabetic from performing endurance exercise, he or she is better advised to take it: endurance exercise improves glucose tolerance and stabilizes blood sugar. These people should simply have their blood glucose levels monitored during the first few weeks of glucosamine sulfate supplementation to identify any blood sugar irregularities that may occur.

Dosages and Additional Natural Supplements

For the treatment of osteoarthritis, the usual daily dosage of glucosamine sulfate is 1,500 mg, which can be taken at one time or in divided doses of 500 mg per dose. Individuals taking diuretic drugs may require an additional 500 mg a day to compensate for their increased excretion rates. Those weighing more than 200 pounds may also be advised to up their dosage to 2,000 mg a day. I generally recommend glucosamine sulfate in a combination formula with other natural anti-inflammatory agents, as outlined below. It should be noted that experts have concluded that adding chondroitin sulfate to glucosamine has shown no benefits beyond glucosamine alone.

While glucosamine sulfate provides the raw material from which cartilage cells make more chondroitin sulfate and hyaluronic acid, it does not directly target the inflammation that is associated with osteoarthritis and joint injury problems. I usually advise patients to add a combination of natural anti-inflammatory herbal agents to their glucosamine sulphate supplement to speed pain relief and reduce joint swelling. You'll often find these herbs already incorporated into manufacturers' glucosamine formulations. Studies indicate that many of these natural agents are as effective as conventional anti-inflammatory drugs with fewer reported adverse side effects. Their availability offers arthritis sufferers another effective treatment for the management of their symptoms and can help eliminate or minimize their reliance on NSAIDS and other synthetic solutions.

Natural anti-inflammatory agents modulate the activity of cyclooxygenase and 5-lipoxygenase, the enzymes that are involved in the inflammatory process. The former enzyme converts arachidonic acid to prostaglandin series –2. PG-2 synthesis is known to produce an inflammatory effect, exacerbating joint pain and irritation. Likewise, 5-lipoxygenase enzyme converts arachidonic acid to leukotriene B4 (LTB-4) within white blood cells, and also contributes to inflammation of the joints. White blood cell count in normal synovial fluid is less than 100 ml on average; however, cellular response rises to 800 ml or more in osteoarthritis and much higher again in rheumatoid diseases. Like many synthetic anti-inflammatory drugs, the active constituents of anti-inflammatory herbs block the activity of the cyclooxygenase and lipoxygenase enzymes, inhibiting the synthesis of pro-inflammatory chemicals, primarily PG-2 and LTB-4 series, and relieving the inflammation and pain associated with arthritis and traumatic joint injuries. Unlike their synthetic counterparts, they have not been shown to cause erosion injury to the intestinal tract, accelerate cartilage destruction, or produce liver and kidney toxicity. For these reasons, the following herbal agents can be considered viable alternatives to conventional anti-inflammatory drugs in a large percentage of arthritic patients and those suffering from other muscle and joint inflammatory conditions. Lower doses may be used if the herbal agent is one of several in a combination formula of anti-inflammatory agents.

Curcumin—the active anti-inflammatory agent found in the spice turmeric. It inhibits the activity of the 5-lipoxygenase and cyclooxygenase enzymes, blocking the synthesis of PG-2 and LTB-4. One large double-blind study demonstrated that curcumin was as effective as the powerful anti-inflammatory drug phenylbutazone in reducing pain, swelling and stiffness in rheumatoid arthritis patients. It has also been helpful in the treatment of post-surgical inflammation. Other studies indicate that curcumin can lower histamine levels and is a potent antioxidant, factors that may contribute to its anti-inflammatory capabilities. For best results, use a 95 percent standardized extract of curcumin derived from turmeric. As a singular agent—that is, if used alone—the recommended daily dosage is 400-600 mg, taken one to three times per day. Side effects are rare, comprising primarily heartburn and esophageal reflux. Curcumin has a mild anti-coagulant effect and caution should exercised if it is combined with powerful anti-coagulant drugs like coumadin, warfarin or plavix, although no drug-nutrient interactions leading to bleeding disorders have been reported in the scientific literature to date.

Boswellia—in clinical studies, the gum resin of the boswellia tree (yielding 70 percent boswellic acids) has improved symptoms in patients with osteoarthritis and rheumatoid arthritis. Research indicates that boswellic acids inhibit the 5-lipoxygenase enzyme in white blood cells. As a singular agent the usual dosage is 150 mg, taken one to three times per day. Boswellia appears to have no significant side effects or drug-nutrient interactions of concern.

White willow bark extract—provides anti-inflammatory phenolic glycosides, such as salicin, which have proven effective in the treatment of arthritis, back pain, and other joint inflammatory conditions. These phenolic glycosides inhibit cyclooxygenase, blocking the production of PG-2 and exert a mild painkilling effect. Unlike aspirin (synthetic acetylsalicylic acid or ASA), naturally occurring salicin does not increase the risk of bleeding disorders. White willow extract is slower-acting than ASA, but its effects last longer. The usual dosage is 20 to 40 mg of salicin, one to three times per day (note that 100 mg of white willow extract at a 15 percent standardized grade of salicin content yields 15 mg of salicin per dosage). Side effects are rare, but include nausea, headache and digestive upset. Contraindications may include conditions where ASA is also contraindicated, such as gout, diabetes, hemophilia, kidney disease, active peptic ulcer, glucose-6-phosphate dehydrogenase deficiency, and possibly asthma. However, the salicin content in a single dosage of white willow extract is very low compared to the acetylsalicylic acid content of ASA (15 mg vs. 320 mg); thus, these conditions may not be absolute contraindications for the use of white willow bark extract. Besides salicin, white willow extract contains other phenolic glycosides known to possess anti-inflammatory properties.

Ginger root extract—contains oleo-resins that have shown clinical benefits in the management of various arthritic and muscle inflammation problems, including rheumatoid arthritis, osteoarthritis, and myalgias. The active constituents are gingerols which inhibit the cyclooxygenase and lipoxygenase enzymes. The usual dosage is 500 mg, one to three times daily, standardized to five percent gingerol content. Side effects are rare, but include heartburn and digestive upset. It should not be given to patients with gallstones.

Bromelain—contains anti-inflammatory enzymes that suppress the inflammation and pain of rheumatoid and osteoarthritis, sports injuries, and other joint inflammatory conditions. Bromelain inhibits the cyclooxygenase enzyme, suppressing the synthesis of PG-2. Bromelain also helps to break down fibrin, thereby minimizing local swelling. The usual dosage is 400 mg, one to three times per day. Bromelain may inhibit platelet clotting and so boost the effects of anticoagulant drugs such as warfarin and coumadin; bleeding time should be monitored by a physician if it is used in cases where these drugs are also taken.

Quercetin—is a bioflavonoid compound that blocks the release of histamine and other pro-inflammatory enzymes at minimum doses of 1,000 to 1,500 mg per day. Although human studies with arthritic patients have yet to be undertaken, anecdotal and experimental evidence is strong for this application. There are no known side effects or drug-nutrient interactions for quercetin. I have used and recommended quercetin in a formula with glucosamine, methyl sulfonyl methane and bromelain enzymes, and have been very impressed with the ability of this combination to relieve arthritic pain more quickly than glucosamine sulfate alone.

Methyl Sulfonyl Methane—MSM is a natural sulfur-containing compound that is produced by the human body and is found in limited quantities in certain foods, such as fruits, vegetables, and meats. MSM ingested in higher doses as a supplement produces anti-inflammatory effects and helps support the integrity of joint cartilage. It has pain-relieving properties and has been used to treat a wide variety of muscle and joint inflammatory conditions. Studies suggest that it may also inhibit the formation of scar tissue around joints and slow the degeneration of cartilage in cases of osteoarthritis. When used on its own the usual dosage is 1,500 to 3,000 mg per day; however, a daily dosage of 200 to 400 mg per day can be beneficial if taken in conjunction with glucosamine sulfate and other natural anti-inflammatory agents. MSM is a very safe substance and is not associated with any drug-nutrient interactions. Its rare side effects may include stomach upset, headache, or more frequent bowel movements.

Devil's claw—contains the anti-inflammatory agent harpogoside. Devil's claw has demonstrated its effectiveness in the management of low back pain and is a traditional anti-inflammatory among many southern African tribes. The usual dosage is 100 to 400 mg, one to three times per day. The only consistently reported side effect is mild and infrequent digestive upset. It is contraindicated in patients with active gastric ulcers (may increase gastric acid secretion) and in patients taking warfarin or coumadin, due to its anticoagulant effects.

A number of companies manufacture single and combination natural anti-inflammatory supplement products that meet the dosage and standardized grade criteria that I have outlined in this section. In conjunction with the use of glucosamine sulphate, these anti-inflammatory agents are a natural, safe, and effective means to help reduce the inflammation and pain associated with osteoarthritis and other joint inflammatory conditions.

For patients with low-grade osteoarthritic symptoms I recommend the use of a supplement that contains glucosamine sulfate, MSM, quercetin, and bromelain enzymes. For patients with more advanced osteoarthritic conditions, I suggest that they add to these a supplement that contains a combination of turmeric (curcumin), boswellia, white willow bark, and ginger.

For patients with rheumatoid arthritis, lupus, other autoimmune inflammatory conditions, tendonitis, bursitis, and joint or muscle inflammation, I recommend the combination of turmeric (curcumin), boswellia, white willow bark, and ginger only, as there appears to be no benefit from glucosamine for primarily inflammatory conditions.

7. Brain Support After 50: CDP-Choline, Phosphatidylserine, Acetyl-L-Carnitine, Bacopa Monnieri, and Huperzine A

One of the cruelest fates is that of the individual who has taken care to stay in good physical condition well into his sixties, seventies, or eighties, only to develop senile dementia, Alzheimer's disease, or debilitating loss of mental capacity while otherwise healthy. According to the U.S. National Institute on Aging, Alzheimer's disease currently affects approximately six to eight percent of all

North Americans over the age of 65 and 47 percent of those over the age of 85. Many of us have witnessed the devastating emotional trauma of these conditions for the afflicted and for their families and friends, and many of us fear this late-life scenario above all others.

Spurred by the advancing years of the baby boomer cohort, anti-aging research has made significant recent progress in understanding long-term brain function. Among the areas of investigation is the influence of natural agents when taken as nutritional supplements, and here researchers have made important discoveries that promise the possibility of slowing or reversing the age-related changes that make us susceptible to memory loss and diminished mental acuity.

How the Brain Ages

There are two main processes at work in the aging of the brain. The first involves the damage to brain cells caused over a lifetime by free radicals. As described earlier, the brain is consuming at least 10 percent of the body's oxygen for energy production at any given moment. This high utilization of oxygen gives rise to oxygen free radicals, which are known to damage brain cells and are suspected of encouraging the formation of the amyloid protein that promotes the development and progression of Alzheimer's disease. The older you are, the greater your brain's cumulative exposure to free radicals and the more extensive the brain cell damage or destruction.

In Step 2 of this book, I suggested that you can protect your brain with the help of a daily high-potency multivitamin that is enriched with antioxidants such as vitamin E, beta-carotene, and vitamin C. Supplementation with melatonin may also be prudent after the age of 40. Lifetime antioxidant supplementation is emerging as a key step in preventing mental deterioration and is the first measure to adopt to preserve functional brain cells as you age.

The second component of brain aging is a decline in the formation of certain brain chemicals known as neurotransmitters, the substances that allow the transfer of impulses from nerve to nerve or nerve to muscle. For instance, after a certain age it appears that the body is programmed to make less of the enzyme necessary for the creation of acetylcholine, the critical brain chemical that is responsible for memory and recall ability. After the age of 60 there is often a significant drop in acetylcholine synthesis. If the decline is severe enough, the result is progressive memory loss and other manifestations of cognitive dysfunction.

It's now known that specific natural supplements can help boost the body's acetylcholine levels. I recommend that after age 50 you incorporate a brain support nutritional supplement into your anti-aging regimen. Here are the nutrients that have been shown to help combat age-related memory loss, cognitive decline, and failing mental acuity.

CDP-choline

CDP-choline (cytidine 5-diphosphocholine or citidinediphospho-choline or citicholine) is a recently discovered nutrient that has proven effective in the management of senile dementia, Alzheimer's disease, and Parkinson's disease.

As described above, choline is one of the essential building blocks of the brain chemical acetylcholine.

In addition to its ability to increase the synthesis of acetyl-choline and other important brain chemicals, CDP-choline contributes to the structure of the outer skin, or membranes, of brain cells, the sites of impulse transfers across the brain. In human trials, supplementation has been effective in cases of senile cognitive impairment, slowing the progression of Alzheimer's disease and Parkinson's disease. In experimental settings, it has increased levels of noradrenaline and dopamine in the central nervous system, two chemicals essential to many cognitive and unconscious brain functions. It also hastens the resorption of cerebral swelling in experimental models. In studies of patients with head trauma, CDP-choline accelerated the recovery from post-traumatic coma and the recuperation of walking ability. Its use reduced the hospital stay of these patients and improved the cognitive and memory disturbances common to post-concussion syndrome.

CDP-choline is well tolerated by patients. No serious side effects have occurred in any of the groups treated with doses in the range of 1,000 mg per day. Toxicology studies likewise indicate that it is a safe intervention, with no adverse effects on the brain function. It is the most reliable form of choline supplementation available to support the brain's synthesis of the memory chemical acetylcholine.

Phosphatidylserine

Phosphatidylserine is a fatty, waxy substance in the body that supports the integrity and fluidity of nerve cell membranes. Low brain levels of phosphatidylserine are associated with impaired cognitive function and depression among the elderly, and in Italy, Scandinavia, and other parts of Europe, phosphatidylserine supplementation is widely used to help address these conditions in the aged. In addition, the serine portion of phosphatidylserine can be converted by the brain into choline, thereby contributing to acetylcholine synthesis.

Numerous studies involving elderly patients (65 to 93 years) with moderate to severe senility, including Alzheimer's patients and depressed elderly patients, have demonstrated significant improvement in memory, behaviour, mood states, and cognitive function with phosphatidylserine supplementation of 100 mg three times daily.

Most of these studies used bovine-derived phosphatidylserine, a product that has since been withdrawn because of the risk of Creutzfeld-Jacob or "mad cow" disease. Today the majority of phosphatidylserine products are derived from soy, but there have been few cognitive function studies so far using this source of phosphatidylserine. Soy and bovine-derived phosphatidylserine are not chemically identical; however, preliminary animal studies show that soy-derived phosphatidylserine does have positive effects on brain function similar to that of bovine-derived, and it is undoubtedly a safer substance. No significant side effects or adverse reactions have been noted with its use, other than mild gastrointestinal distress on rare occasions.

Acetyl-L-Carnitine

Acetyl-L-Carnitine (ALC) is a nutrient produced by the body, with high concentrations found in the brain, muscles, liver, kidney, and testes. It is thought that the decline in ALC synthesis by the body after age 50 is a major contributor to age-related cognitive impairment and possibly Alzheimer's disease.

Double-blind clinical trials showed improvement in such patients when ALC was administered at daily dosages ranging from 1,000 to 2,000 mg per day. ALC has been shown to be nontoxic and extremely safe for human use. Rare side effects include skin rash, nausea, vomiting, and agitation.

Bacopa Monnieri

The leaf of bacopa, or water hyssop, has been used in Ayurveda, traditional Hindu medicine, since the sixth century to help improve mental performance. Its active ingredients enhance nerve transmission and are potent antioxidants.

Currently, bacopa is being used and studied as a natural substance to strengthen memory and general cognition and to help control epilepsy. The data suggests that bacopa supplementation can increase learning ability in laboratory animals, while human studies have provided evidence that it may improve intellectual activity in children and memory and mental performance in adults. In one study reported by *Psychopharmacology* in 2001, healthy volunteers were given bacopa monnieri supplementation (300 mg per day) or a placebo, with follow-up neuropsychological testing performed at weeks 5 and 12. Compared to the placebo group, the subjects given bacopa significantly improved their speed of visual information processing, learning rate, and memory consolidation, and they demonstrated reduced anxiety levels. The researchers concluded that bacopa monnieri may improve higher-order cognitive processes that are dependent on the input of information such as learning and memory. There are no well-known side effects from the use of bacopa monnieri at recommended doses.

Huperzine A

Huperzine A is an alkaloid compound found in low concentrations in a moss from the Lycopodiaceae family. It has been used for centuries in Chinese folk medicine to treat a range of ailments, but in modern times research has focused on its ability to raise brain levels of acetylcholine. When used therapeutically, huperzine A , or hupA, is given as a concentrated extract. Commercially available products contain up to 95 percent hupA concentration.

Huperzine A is rapidly absorbed by the brain, where it acts as a potent inhibitor of the enzyme acetylcholinesterase, which breaks down the memory chemical acetylcholine. A feature of

Alzheimer's disease is reduced concentrations of acetylcholine in specific areas of the brain. Huperzine A supplementation appears to help boost these levels in cases where the condition has not yet advanced to the point of permanent brain cell damage.

Studies show that huperzine A provides a longer-lasting effect than tacrine or doneprizil, drugs which are often prescribed for Alzheimer's disease, and with fewer side effects.

In a 1995 double-blind clinical study of Alzheimer's disease patients by Dr. S.S. Xu and colleagues in China, the group given 200 mcg of huperzine A twice a day for eight weeks demonstrated marked improvement in memory, cognitive, and behavioural functions. It has also been used successfully in a clinical setting in China with approximately 100,000 Alzheimer's and dementia patients. At Beijing's Institute of Mental Health it was tested against fodine, another drug for Alzheimer's disease, in 101 patients with benign senescent forgetfulness. After four weeks of supplementation, 70 percent of the group receiving huperzine A showed improvement in their memory, prompting the researchers to include an additional 111 Alzheimer's patients in the study. Overall, the group receiving hupA demonstrated a 10 percent improvement in the memory quotient over the four-week test period, and significant improvement in other measures of cognitive function. Side effects occurred in only three percent of these patients, the most frequent being dizziness and gastrointestinal symptoms. Other reliable studies undertaken in China showed similar positive results with Alzheimer's patients and favourable comparisons to synthetic drugs.

Side effects associated with huperzine A supplementation are rare at recommended doses, but as mentioned may include dizziness and gastrointestinal symptoms.

Don't Mix Brain Support Supplements with Other Brain Support Medications Without Your Doctor's Consent

Individuals with Alzheimer's disease, dementia, depression, or other mental or psychological ailments who are on medication for these conditions must check with their attending physicians before taking the herbal and accessory nutrients described here.

Combining prescription medications with these supplements can amplify the effects of certain drugs to the point of toxicity and life-threatening crisis.

Do Take Brain Support Supplements Before Age-Related Changes Take Hold

As a measure of prevention, it is advisable to take an all-in-one brain support supplement to combat the body's pre-programmed decline in memory ability and cognitive function. This supplement should be used in conjunction with a high-potency multivitamin and mineral and an essential fatty acid supplement, both of which contain nutrients that also play a vital role in preserving the integrity of brain cells.

An all-in-one brain support supplement that I recommend for anti-aging purposes includes the following ingredients and dosages per capsule:

- CDP-Choline – 50 mg
- Phosphatidylserine – 50 mg
- Huperzine A – 25 mcg
- Bacopa Monnieri – 50 mg (standardized to 20 percent bacosides content)
- Acetyl-L-Carnitine – 150 mg

Take two capsules a day for brain support, beginning between the ages of 50 and 60.

Be Cautious with the Use of Other Brain Support Supplements

There are three other brain support supplements that are considered beneficial in preserving or restoring memory and other aspects of cognitive function, but their potential side effects demand proper monitoring by a qualified health care professional. These supplements are ginkgo biloba, vinpocetine, and dimethylaminoethanol.

Ginkgo biloba extract increases blood flow to the brain and has been known to improve cases of memory loss, Alzheimer's disease, and age-related cognitive decline. Unfortunately, some of its active ingredients produce a powerful anti-coagulant effect, which has caused internal bleeding in several reported cases, including bleeding in the brain.

Vinpocetine is an isolated substance from a plant called lesser periwinkle. Like ginkgo biloba, vinpocetine increases blood flow to the brain and has shown success in patients with Alzheimer's disease, ischemic stroke, dementia and chronic cerebral insufficiency (reduced blood flow to the brain causing disturbances in memory and cognitive function). It too is a strong anti-coagulant with the associated risk of internal bleeding.

Ginkgo biloba and vinpocetine should not be taken by individuals who regularly use other anti-coagualant drugs such as aspirin, coumadin, warfarin, or plavix. As a general rule, these supplements should not be taken without proper monitoring by a doctor, and their indiscriminant use is not advised.

Dimethylaminoethanol (DMAE or Deanol) is a natural product that may increase brain levels of choline. However, clinical trials have brought to light frequent side effects, including drowsiness, confusion, lucid dreams, depression, dull headache, increased tension of the jaw and other muscles, and insomnia. I do not recommend its use at this time.

8. Preserving Libido and Sexual Function: Muira Puama, Tribulus Terrestris, Epimedium, Damiana, and Avena Sativa

One very common aspect of aging that deserves attention for its influence on quality of life after 50 is reduced libido and compromised sexual function in both men and women.

For men, the difficulty is defined as erectile dysfunction, a consistent inability to achieve or maintain an erection sufficient for satisfactory sexual relations. Complete erectile dysfunction is the absolute inability to achieve penetration at any stage of sexual relations. The 2004 Massachusetts Male Aging Study of 1,300 men between the ages of 40 and 70 suggested that just over half of all men in this age group have some degree of erectile dysfunction; five percent of 40-year-olds and 25 percent of 75-year-olds have complete erectile dysfunction. In another study of 216 men aged 40 to 79 who experienced varying degrees of erectile dysfunction, Dr. F.E. Kaiser et al reported that no patient over the age of 70 experienced full erections, even of short duration. This investigation also showed that the most significant alterations in testosterone secretion related to erectile dysfunction and the most significant decline in blood flow to the penis resulting from narrowed arteries occur after the age of 50.

For women, menopause may trigger a loss of interest in sex and introduce physiological changes, such as vaginal dryness, that can make intercourse painful. A 2004 investigation by Dr. J.E. Blumel and fellow researchers concluded that between 40 and 64 years of age, approximately 40 percent of women cease to have sexual relations. Unhappy personal relationships with partners and an absence of partners were both cited, but sexual dysfunction—low sexual desire—was the primary reason given in 49 percent of these cases.

The Causes of Sexual Dysfunction

For men, the age-related decline in testosterone synthesis and secretion is closely associated with reduced libido and erectile dysfunction problems. Between 40 and 70 years of age, the average testosterone level drops by about one percent every year—a significant 30 percent reduction.

Other reasons for male sexual dysfunction include diabetes (due to narrowed arteries, a frequent complication of this disease), atherosclerosis (the buildup of cholesterol plaque on the walls of the arteries, causing reduced blood flow to the erectile tissues of the penis), the use of drugs used in the treatment of depression or psychological disorders or that lower blood pressure, alcohol consumption, and social-psychological factors (lack of attraction, poor relationship with partner, anxiety, depression). Prostate enlargement, and the accompanying lower urinary tract symptoms (LUTS), is another common cause. Men with LUTS have a higher risk of erectile dysfunction than those with no clinically significant prostate enlargement, and they report a higher incidence of ejaculatory loss and painful ejaculation. This is further justification for the use of a prostate support supplement after the age of 40.

Erectile dysfunction can also be attributed to a decrease in vibrotactile sensitivity due to a loss of nerve receptors in the skin of the penis. These receptors register tactile sensations when the penis is touched and transmit pleasurable sexual signals through the nerve pathways that lead to the spinal cord and up to the brain. With age, there are fewer of these receptors, so there can be too little sensory stimulation to produce or sustain an erection through the normal automatic reflex nerve channels.

In women, age-related sexual dysfunction and loss of libido are most strongly linked to the significant drop in estrogen, progesterone, and testosterone that accompanies menopause.

Potentially Risky Treatments

The medical profession has largely approached the treatment of sexual dysfunction and loss of libido with a "topping up" strategy—hormone replacement therapy for women, testosterone replacement for men, and growth hormone injections for both. Also frequently prescribed for both is the administration of extra DHEA (dehydroepiendrosterone), a steroid hormone that the body can convert into testosterone and estrogen. These drugs have been proven effective, no question. However, their use increases the risk of breast cancer, heart disease, and stroke, and may increase the risk of colon and prostate cancer.

Hormone Therapy for Women

As outlined earlier, the use of hormone replacement therapy by women for the management of menopause and to prevent osteoporosis has fallen out of favor since the findings of the Women's Health Initiative Study were made public. As a treatment for sexual dysfunction, it is no less risky.

DHEA Supplementation

DHEA has been used as an agent to help manage menopause in women and andropause in men, and some studies suggest that it can be effective in cases of sexual dysfunction. This steroid hormone is created from cholesterol in the adrenal glands. As we age, blood levels of DHEA decline, providing less of the raw material for testosterone and estrogen synthesis to our reproductive tissues.

Some anti-aging experts have recommended DHEA supplementation beginning between ages 40 and 50 as means of allowing the body to make its own testosterone and estrogen. Thus far, reports of its effectiveness as an anti-aging supplement have been mixed and inconclusive. Although some patients have experienced enhanced sexual performance and libido, experimental evidence suggests that DHEA supplementation may encourage the growth of latent breast cancer and prostate cancer, both known to occur at higher rates in individuals over 50.

Until DHEA can be shown to be a safe intervention in this respect, and I think that is unlikely to happen, I don't recommend it as a treatment option for men with erectile dysfunction problems and loss of libido, or as a libido-enhancing treatment for women

Testosterone Replacement Therapy for Men

Testosterone replacement therapy is a proven method to enhance male sex drive and sexual performance in men with these problems. However, testosterone is also known to foster the growth and spread of detected prostate cancers, and many practitioners are reluctant to prescribe it to maintain sexual virility for fear it may promote the development of undetected prostate cancer cells that otherwise may not have posed a threat.

My view is that any therapy that encourages higher levels of DHT (the male prostate converts testosterone into DHT) in the body is likely to promote the development of prostate cancer. I recommend that men use more natural remedies as their first approach to this problem, as I will outline shortly

Growth Hormone Injections

We'll deal with growth hormone in greater detail in the section that follows this one, but in the context of libido and sexual function, research studies have shown that growth hormone injections and Insulin-like Growth Factor-1 (IGF-1) can help both men and women.

Remember that higher circulating levels of growth hormone in the bloodstream stimulate higher secretions of IGF-1 from the liver. It is IGF-1 that actually produces the physiological effects of growth hormone. Injecting either growth hormone or IGF-1 will produce a rise in IGF-1 blood levels. It may be the case, though, that these injections will raise IGF-1 levels into a range that promotes the development of undetected cancers. At the moment, no one can identify the precise optimal level of IGF-1 that will reverse aging and enhance sexual performance without increasing cancer risk. The medical evidence is consistent that excess growth hormone, whether from injections or caused naturally (for example, by the condition acromegaly, in which the pituitary gland secretes excess growth hormone) is associated with an increased risk of colon cancer. More recently it has been shown that various cancer cells increase their synthesis of IGF-1, fostering their own growth and replication, when stimulated by growth hormone.

Consequently, using growth hormone injections as a treatment for sexual dysfunction is not without safety concerns. It appears that the growth hormone secretagogue is a safer choice, in that they do not elevate IGF-1 levels above 275 to 300 ng/ml. That is a level that has not been associated with increased cancer risk. Preliminary reports suggest that secretagogue supplements can improve sexual function and libido in men and women and can be considered for this purpose by individuals who have no history of personal cancer.

Viagra

The prescription drug Viagra has gained tremendous popularity for its ability to reverse erectile dysfunction and improve sexual performance in men. Viagra works by increasing the amount of nitric oxide in the blood vessels that feed the erectile tissues of the penis. This opens up blood flow to the erectile tissues, supporting erection ability and endurance. Yet even this miracle medication is not without hazards.

Viagra is not to be taken by men who have heart disease (angina, congestive heart failure, or patients taking multi-drug anti-hypertensive agents), kidney or liver disease, or who are taking the drugs erythromycin or cimetidine. These precautions are in place because Viagra can cause a precipitous decline in blood pressure during the 24 hours after ingestion, at which point nitroglycerine drugs must also be avoided.

In 2001 a research team from Cedars-Sinai Medical Center in Los Angles analyzed reports of Viagra's ill effects collected by the Food and Drug Administration. In 1,473 serious adverse events reported, 522 men had died, most of cardiovascular causes. The majority of deaths (70 percent) were associated with the standard Viagra dosage of 50 milligrams; two-thirds of the victims had taken Viagra within five hours of their deaths being reported; and most of the dead were younger than 65 and had no reported heart disease risk factors.

The study confirmed the well-documented danger of combining nitrate use with Viagra. Of the 90 patients who were on nitrates and taking Viagra, 68 percent died, and another 20 percent suffered non-fatal heart attacks. (Viagra's manufacturer, Pfizer, officially discourages mixing Viagra and organic nitrates, such as nitroglycerin.) But a whopping 88 percent of deaths occurred in patients who were not taking nitrates. That led investigators to speculate that there are significant numbers who are subject to other harmful effects from Viagra. More recently these effects have been linked to increased risk of stroke and other cardiovascular reactions which can lead to ruptured atherosclerotic plaques within blood vessels, thrombus formation, and headaches. The speed of the symptoms leading to death and the fact that 88 percent of the fatalities were first-time users suggest that some individuals are highly susceptible.

Safe, Natural Herbal Remedies that Enhance Libido and Sexual Function in Men and Women

For many centuries cultures around the world have used natural herbal agents to enhance libido and sexual function. A number of them have shown impressive results in modern-day clinical trials of human subjects with known problems. Researchers have identified the active constituents or the mechanisms at work in these herbal products, and tests for toxicity, side effects and potential drug-nutrient interactions have been established for most to ensure that they can be used in a safe, effective, and responsible manner. A number of studies have shown that combining some of these herbal agents into one supplement product offers greater positive effects on sexual function than a single sexual-enhancement herb alone.

At the end of this section I'll outline the herbal combination product that I recommend. However, let's first get acquainted with these individual herbal agents.

Muira Puama (Potency Wood)

Muira puama extract is made from the root of a shrub native to Brazil, long used as a powerful aphrodisiac and nerve-stimulant in South American folk medicine. Early European explorers returned home with the muira puama plant, and it has been used in European herbal medicine for centuries since. In England, muira puama is listed in the British Herbal Pharmacopoeia as a treatment for impotence and dysentery.

Two clinical studies conducted at the Institute of Sexology in France in 1990 and 2000 showed that muira puama extract can reverse erectile dysfunction in a high percentage of men within a two-week period: 85 percent of subjects reported an enhanced libido; 100 percent, increased frequency of intercourse; and 90 percent, an improved ability to maintain an erection.

Results of a 2000 study, also conducted at the Institute of Sexology and involving 202 women with low sex drive, demonstrated that a combination supplement product containing muira puama and ginkgo biloba (Herbal vX), taken for one month, improved libido and other aspects of sexual function in 65 percent of the participants. The researchers stated that statistically significant improvements occurred in frequency of sexual desire, sexual intercourse and sexual fantasies, as well as in intensity of sexual desires, excitement of fantasies, ability to reach orgasm, and intensity of orgasm.

Its precise mechanism of action remains unknown, though it appears to enhance both the psychological and physical aspects of sexual function. The usual dosage is 1,000 to 1,500 mg per day. Muira puama has not been associated with any significant side effects or toxicity.

Tribulus Terrestris (Puncture Vine)

Tribulus terrestris is a natural herb, commonly known as puncture vine, that has been used for hundreds of years in Europe. In Ayurvedic medicine, it is known as a tonic for treating genito-urinary troubles and impotence. In China, tribulus is prescribed as a treatment for high blood pressure and angina and for a variety of liver and kidney conditions. In Bulgaria, it is taken by men and women as an antidote to infertility and by Olympic athletes who claim to have used high doses to increase muscle development. (The research data to support this claim has never been revealed to exercise physiologists in the West.)

One of the most consistent findings related to tribulus is its ability to enhance sexual performance in men and stimulate libido in men and women, thanks in part to its hormonal effects. In animal and human male studies, tribulus supplementation can raise testosterone levels by 30 to 40 percent, the result of an increase in the release of luteinizing hormone (LH) from the pituitary gland, which in turn increases testosterone production in the testes. These hormonal alterations can also step up sperm production and motility, hence its application as a treatment for infertility. One human study showed that LH blood levels rose 72 percent after supplementation with 750 mg per day of tribulus terrestris (standardized to 45 percent saponin content) and that free testosterone rose by 41 percent in male subjects. (Free testosterone is not bound to a protein carrier in the bloodstream, making it more available for use by the cells and more potent than bound testosterone.)

A second beneficial feature of tribulus terrestris is its ability to increase the release of nitric oxide from the lining of blood vessels and nerves that supply blood flow to the penis. This results in a relaxation of the blood vessels, which in turn allows greater engorgement of blood within the erectile tissues and a firmer and longer lasting erection. Improvements in erectile dysfunction often occur on the first day of use or within the first few days of use, which is too soon to be the result of a rise in testosterone levels.

In general, human studies involving male subjects, as well as anecdotal evidence, indicate that tribulus terrestris supplementation can increase libido, frequency, and strength of erections; increase sperm count and motility; and shorten the time between erections. Its active ingredients have not been completely identified; however, much research indicates that its furostanol saponins are likely a principle ingredient. Studies yielding the best results for men have used tribulus terrestris supplements that are standardized to contain 40 to 45 percent steroidal saponins.

Among women, tribulus increases the concentration of hormones including estradiol, with testosterone being very slightly influenced, which is associated with improved sexual function and libido. It is also thought to increase clitorial blood flow, adding to sensitivity and sexual responsiveness. A 1988 study by Dr. P. Tabakova and fellow researchers in Bulgaria showed that tribulus terrestris supplementation in women improved libido and sexual function in 66 percent of subjects with reported low sex drive and sexual dysfunction problems.

Tribulus terrestris is not only a safe, natural agent to improve and restore male and female sexual virility, but its daily use is associated with a number of significant anti-aging and disease-prevention effects. In China, large clinical trials with patients have shown it to be effective in the treatment of angina, with no adverse side effects or damage to the circulatory system, kidneys, or liver. Other researchers have found that it reduces high blood pressure, lowers blood cholesterol, and acts as a natural anti-inflammatory, performing in a similar fashion to drugs like Celebrex and Vioxx but without the intestinal tract irritation of aspirin or ibuprofen.

In addition, tribulus terrestris contains beta-sitosterol, which, as we've seen, promotes male prostate health by reducing the production of inflammatory prostaglandin hormones and by inhibiting the enzyme that converts testosterone into DHT, a known contributor to prostate enlargement and prostate cancer. Its steroidal compounds can improve immune function due to their antibacterial and antiviral properties, which has led to its use as a treatment for herpes and other viral infections such as flus and the common cold.

For all of these reasons, tribulus terrestris an attractive supplement for men and women over the age of 50. No adverse effects to the central nervous or cardiovascular systems were noted in any of the clinical studies using tribulus terrestris and no toxicity or deviations in blood count were observed. There are no known negative effects when tribulus is used as a dietary supplement. The usual dosage to preserve or restore sexual virility is 750 to 1,500 mg per day.

Damiana (Tunera aphrodisiaca)

Damiana is found throughout Mexico, Central America, and the Caribbean. Its Latin name, *Tunera aphrodisiaca,* advertises its reputation. In the Netherlands it is renowned for its sexual enhancing qualities and positive effect on the reproductive organs, and it has been used as an aphrodisiac in North America since 1874.

The pharmacology of the plant suggests that its alkaloids may have hormone-like effects, plus it increases the sensitivity of the genital organs by very slightly irritating the urethra and possibly other tissues that line the reproductive tract.

It is usually included in sex-enhancement supplements along with other virility herbs. A typical capsule contains 200 to 300 mg of damiana in formulations that are usually taken three times per day or three capsules all at once.

Epimedium (Horny Goat Weed)

Epimedium is a plant common to the grazing and farming regions of China. Many years ago, Chinese farmers noticed that their goats became much friskier and copulated much more frequently after grazing on this plant (hence its common name, "horny goat weed"). Epimedium is an important supplement in traditional Chinese medicine, where it is considered a powerful sex stimulant, and it's now gaining popularity in the western world.

Epimedium's leaves contain a variety of healthful flavonoids, polysaccharides, and sterols, as well as an alkaloid called magnaflorine. Its exact mechanism of action is still something of a mystery, but it has been successful in boosting sexual desire, aiding erectile function, and fighting fatigue.

As a sexual-enhancement herb, the standardized grade of epimedium should contain 10 percent icariin flavonoids, usually providing 100 mg of epimedium per capsule. Epimedium is often included as an ingredient in a multi-herbal sexual enhancement formulation. There have been no reports of adverse side effects associated with the use of epimedium at recommended dosages.

Avena Sativa (Wild Oat)

Avena sativa, or wild oat, is a grass which is cultivated as an edible grain. The parts of the herb typically used for supplementation purposes—the seeds and the stem—contain many active constituents, including saponins, flavonoids, and alkaloids, as well as vitamins, minerals, and other nutrients. Avena sativa supplementation nourishes the nerves, increasing tactile sensations in the genital area. In a 1986 study conducted at the Institute for Advanced Study of Human Sexuality in San Francisco, California, subjects took 300 mg of avena sativa three days per week for six weeks. The 20 men and 20 women in the study ranged from 22 to 64 years of age. The men reported a 22 percent increase in genital sensation and a 36 percent increase in frequency of orgasms, while the women experienced a 15 percent increase in genital sensation and a 29 percent increase in the frequency of orgasms.

Avena sativa is nontoxic and not associated with any adverse side effects or drug-nutrient interactions. Like the others, it is often included with several herbal sexual-enhancement agents in a single supplement product.

Virility Herbs with Questionable Safety Profiles

There are other natural agents that are acknowledged to be effective in cases of erectile and sexual dysfunction, but their potential side effects require care and informed caution if they are to be consumed safely. I strongly advise against the casual use of any of the following herbal agents and support their prescribed use only in special circumstances where their administration and effects can be monitored by a physician.

Yohimbe

Yohimbine, an alkaloid compound derived from the yohimbe plant, increases blood flow to erectile tissue through its direct effects on the nervous system. However, yohimbine produces several undesirable and dangerous side effects, among them anxiety, panic attacks, hallucinations, high blood pressure, rapid heart rate, dizziness, headaches, and skin flushing, and it can aggravate kidney problems and existing psychological disturbances.

Although it is an FDA-approved treatment for impotence, it is classified as an unsafe herb that should be taken only under medical supervision. Many yohimbe products sold over the counter do not contain sufficient yohimbine content to be effective: authentic yohimbe bark contains six percent yohimbine content, and this is the effective standardized grade. Yohimbe supplementation should not be used unless prescribed by a physician.

Ginkgo Biloba Extract

Ginkgo biloba extract (GBE) has a very high success rate in the treatment of erectile dysfunction attributed to poor blood flow as a result of atherosclerosis or diabetes. In two major studies, men with erectile dysfunction who failed to respond to papavernine (a drug injected to produce an erection) or other drugs that improve blood flow demonstrated a marked positive response to the oral ingestion of GBE at 60 or 80 mg, three times per day, in trials lasting six to 18 months. GBE is known to open up blood vessels and inhibit the coagulation of the blood, hence its ability to increase blood flow to the erectile tissues of the penis. Women who used the herbal sexual-enhancement product Herbal vX in an open trial reported significant increases in sexual desire, sexual intercourse, and sexual fantasies, as well improved ability to reach orgasm and intensity of orgasm. Herbal vX contains muira puama and ginkgo biloba.

However, a daily dosage of 180 to 240 mg of GBE, which were the dosages used in the studies on male subjects with erectile dysfunction problems, acts as a powerful anti-coagulant. There have been several reported cases of bleeding into the brain in patients who have used GBE either alone or in combination with other anti-coagulant agents—such as aspirin, NSAIDs, coumadin, warfarin, or Plavix—at doses as low as 40 mg, once to three times per day. I do not recommend that GBE be included as a standard ingredient in an anti-aging sexual virility supplement for men or women. In more extreme cases of sexual impotence or low sex drive, GBE may be used as an additional supplement, provided a physician is consulted to monitor bleeding time as a precaution against potential bleeding disorders. To be effective, GBE extracts must be standardized to contain 24 percent flavone glycosides and six percent terpenes.

Ginseng

In men, panax ginseng increases sperm count and motility, plasma total and free testosterone, dihydrotestosterone, follicle stimulating hormone, and leutinizing hormone. An in vitro study suggests that ginseng may relax the corpus cavernosum by releasing nitric oxide, which improves blood flow and facilitates an erection. A double-blind clinical study showed that ginseng extract supplementation at a daily dosage of 1,800 mg per day for three months helped improve libido and the ability to maintain and erection in men with erectile dysfunction.

Ginseng is an ingredient in a sex-enhancing product known as Argimax for Women, which also contains ginkgo biloba extract, damiana, L-arginine, and multivitamins and minerals. In a four-week clinical trial of 77 females over age 21, subjects reported improved overall satisfaction with sex life in 73.5 percent of users, compared to 37.2 percent in the placebo group. Notable improvements were identified in sexual desire, reduction of vaginal dryness, frequency of sexual intercourse and orgasm, and clitorial sensation. No significant side effects were noted.

To what degree ginseng contributed to these results is unknown. It has been reported to interfere with medications that affect mood disorders (antidepressant drugs, for example), causing symptoms of mania. It may also interact with anti-coagulant drugs and digoxin. On its own, ginseng has been known to cause breast tenderness, postmenopausal vaginal bleeding, and menstrual disorders, due to its hormone-like effects.

In my view ginseng should not be a standard ingredient in libido and sexual-enhancement supplement products, but as is the case with ginkgo biloba, it may be added as a supplement in specific circumstances where there are no drug-nutrient interactions of concern and proper monitoring of potential side effects is in place.

Cordyceps

Cordyceps is a rare mushroom that grows on caterpillars found at high altitudes in Tibet and China and is one of the most valued medicinal agents in traditional Chinese medicine. It is used as a general longevity tonic, to enhance vitality and endurance, and as a treatment for asthma, bronchitis, and kidney disease. Some sex-enhancement supplements include cordyceps for its enhancement of blood flow to the body's extremities, including the sex organs. Cordyceps is one of three ingredients in a product called Venix, a combination of ginkgo biloba extract, cordyceps, and L-arginine. In a randomized, placebo-controlled clinical trial, Venix was taken by 46 male and female participants for 12 weeks. Overall, male subjects reported a 34 percent improvement in sexual function and libido enhancement. There was no notable change in women.

In my view, cordyceps should not be included in a standard anti-aging sexual-enhancement supplement due to its anti-coagulant properties, which may increase the risk of a bleeding disorder. It may also interfere with the function of certain antidepressant medications. Its use requires proper monitoring of bleeding time; it should not be taken by individuals who are using antidepressant or mood-altering medications. Like ginkgo biloba, ginseng, and L-arginine, cordyceps may be used by certain individuals in exceptional cases, provided proper monitoring is in place.

L-Arginine

L-arginine is an amino acid that serves many purposes in the body. At high dosages it can be converted into nitric oxide, which dilates certain blood vessels and improves blood flow. In a preliminary trial, men with erectile dysfunction were given 2,800 mg of arginine, per day, for two weeks. Six of the 15 men noted improvement in erection and sexual performance ability. In a larger, double-blind clinical trial, men with erectile dysfunction were given 1,670 mg of arginine per day, with a significant success rate compared to the placebo group.

Arginine is an ingredient in the sexual-enhancement supplements Argimax for Women and Venix, both of which have shown impressive results in the improvement of female and male sexual performance and libido. The cautionary note is that taken in high doses, arginine too appears to act as a blood thinner and may increase the risk of a bleeding disorder. Here again, I don't recommend its use without appropriate monitoring, and it should not be taken in conjunction with anti-coagulant drugs. Arginine supplementation has also been known to promote outbreaks of herpes lesions such as cold sores and genital herpes in afflicted individuals.

The Standard Anti-Aging Libido and Sex-Enhancement Supplement for Men and Women

For men and women who experience reduced sex drive or compromised sexual function as they age—usually beginning between ages 40 and 50—I recommend a standard herbal combination libido and sexual-enhancement supplement that contains the following ingredients in a single capsule:

- Tribulus terrestris – 250 mg (standardized to 40 to 45 percent saponin content)
- Muira puama – 280 mg
- Epimedium (horny goat weed) – 100 mg
- Damiana – 50 mg
- Avena sativa (wild oat) – 50 mg

Take one capsule three times per day with meals, or all three capsules at once with a meal. In some cases individuals may need to double this dosage at the beginning, cutting back to the standard daily dosage once the product begins to work for them. In addition, the use of melatonin or a growth hormone secretagogue (for example, Meditropin), one hour before bedtime, may also be beneficial.

9. Melatonin: A Versatile and Powerful Anti-Aging and Disease-Prevention Hormone

Melatonin molecules have been found in every animal and plant species, from the most primitive one-celled algae to complex *homo sapiens*. In every organism, melatonin's molecular structure is identical—a rare occurrence in nature—and its production pattern is the same: a secretion cycle that repeats itself roughly every 24 hours, with output higher at night than during the day. In humans, it acts as a hormone, a neurotransmitter, an antioxidant, and an immune system stimulator. This versatility accounts for its many profound effects on our health.

Melatonin is made in the brain's pineal gland from serotonin, a mood-enhancing, appetite-suppressing brain chemical. Daylight stimulates the production of serotonin: the more sunlight entering the pupil of the eye, the greater the synthesis of serotonin and the better we feel. Darkness allows serotonin to be converted into melatonin. At night, the body produces up to ten times more melatonin than in daytime, with levels peaking around two or three o'clock in the morning. The darker the room, the more melatonin secreted. In the morning, exposure to light shuts down melatonin production.

The body's production of melatonin begins to decline after puberty. A 40-year-old generates approximately 60 percent less melatonin than a 10-year-old; by age 70, melatonin levels may be undetectable. The regular use of certain drugs such as aspirin, ibuprofen, and beta-blockers (drugs designed to control high blood pressure) also contributes to lower melatonin levels. This decline in melatonin synthesis and secretion is considered to be a significant factor in accelerated aging, increased risk of certain cancers, dementia, Alzheimer's disease, and weakened immune systems. Many anti-aging experts recommend the ingestion of a melatonin supplement by age 50 to help combat aging, boost immune system function, reduce cancer and heart disease risk—and enjoy better-quality sleep.

Melatonin for a Good Night's Sleep

As a neurotransmitter, melatonin is best known for its ability to elevate mood, similar to serotonin, and to induce sleep in persons with insomnia or interrupted sleep. We sleep roughly 16 hours a day as infants, eight hours in adolescence, seven hours as adults, and less than six hours in our geriatric years. As reported in the

British Medical Journal in 1994, the quality of sleep in elderly individuals is proportional to the amount of melatonin secreted by their pineal glands. A lower output is strongly associated with shortened sleep duration and less deep-level sleep. Delta sleep, the deepest and most restorative, is prevalent in childhood, decreases at puberty, and declines progressively after age 30. As we get older we often feel the need to rest more, but we rarely wake completely rejuvenated and re-energized in the morning as we did in our youth.

As a sleep aid, melatonin is safer than traditional sleeping pills, which come with a host of side effects and toxicity problems. Research shows that, taken at the right dosage one hour before bedtime, it helps individuals fall asleep more quickly and remain in the deeper levels of sleep for longer periods. (This is one of the ways that melatonin strengthens the immune system, which is known to be most active during delta sleep.) There is no morning drowsiness; instead, subjects report feelings of wellbeing throughout the day. It is nontoxic, and leading melatonin researchers, such as Dr. Russell Reiter, have established that it can be used with a high degree of safety.

Melatonin and Breast and Prostate Cancer Prevention

The age-related decline in melatonin secretion may allow breast cancer and prostate cancer to develop more easily. Conversely, the presence of melatonin may help ward off these cancers.

A review of human studies published in 2003 in *Critical Reviews in Oncology/Hematology* pointed to the number of investigations that showed an increased risk of breast cancer in women who are regularly deprived of darkness at night, such as night shift workers, flight attendants, and radio and telegraph operators. There was a decreased risk of breast cancer reported in women who were blind and who routinely had higher circulating levels of melatonin. (Light does not suppress melatonin secretion in the blind to the degree that it does in sighted individuals.) The review noted that this evidence is consistent with the findings of studies in rodents whereby exposure to constant light or removal of the pineal gland, both of which suppress melatonin levels, stimulates the development of breast cancer. Treatment of these animals with melatonin under the same circumstances inhibited breast cancer development.

Experimental studies show that melatonin has an anti-estrogen effect on reproductive tissues, toning down the overstimulation and rapid replication of breast cells caused by estrogen. Others have demonstrated that melatonin can reduce the replication rate of human breast cancer cells by 50 to 75 percent when those cells are exposed to alternating levels of melatonin, mimicking day and night secretion patterns.

It appears to work in a similar fashion as tamoxifen, the widely used drug that prevents the recurrence of breast cancer and its metastases in women who have estrogen-receptor-positive breast cancer. In fact, experimental and human studies have demonstrated that melatonin can enhance the ability of tamoxifen to inhibit breast cancer cell replication. In one trial, Dr. Paolo Lissoni of the division of oncological radiotherapy at Gerardo Hospital in Milan, Italy, combined tamoxifen therapy and melatonin supplementation (20 mg twice per day) in the treatment of his breast cancer patients. Four out of the fourteen women experienced a 50 percent or greater reduction in the size of their tumors. Eight showed no further progression in tumor size, and only two failed to respond to the treatment. These were better results than the typical outcomes associated with tamoxifen use alone. Larger studies of this kind are currently underway to better understand the usefulness of melatonin as a cancer therapy agent.

From the standpoint of prevention, the evidence suggests that melatonin may protect against breast cancer in several ways. First, as mentioned, it counters the effects of estrogen on breast cells, slowing the rate of cell division and reducing the chances that a cancer cell will develop. Second, should a cancer cell develop in the breast, melatonin will inhibit its ability to divide and spread. And third, melatonin enhances the effectiveness of the immune system's natural killer cells to seek out and destroy cancer cells before they can take hold. As a bonus, melatonin is a powerful antioxidant that helps prevent free radical damage to all body tissues, including the DNA of breast cells.

Like breast cancer patients, males with diagnosed prostate cancer exhibit low blood levels of melatonin. It's not yet been determined if these low levels increase the risk of prostate and breast cancer development or if the cancers cause the reduction in melatonin. However, with respect to prostate cancer, the results of studies published between 2000 and 2002 by Drs. A. Rimler, S.W. Siu, S.C Xi, and M.M. Marelli showed that melatonin inhibits the growth and replication of the most commonly encountered human prostate cancer cells in experimental conditions.

These findings may explain the outcome of an important case study reported in 1987 by Dr. Lissoni, an Italian researcher who has used melatonin in some clinical trials. In a confirmed case of localized prostate cancer, melatonin supplementation at six mg per day reduced the prostate specific antigen blood level (PSA) from 30 to four within six months. PSA is an indirect marker of the activity of a prostate tumor. A normal PSA range is between zero and four. In 2003, a similar case study was reported by Dr. S.Y. Shiu in the *Journal of Pineal Research*. It showed that the administration of five mg of melatonin per day blocked the further rise in PSA levels in a patient with prostate cancer and stabilized the progression of his disease after standard medical interventions (castration and hormone therapy) had failed to prevent its recurrence.

The Lissoni and Shiu results suggest that it may be advantageous for men who are in the watchful waiting stage of prostate cancer to take five to 10 mg of melatonin one hour before bedtime every night, in addition to doubling or tripling the dosage of the prostate supplement formula, described in Step 3 of this book, on protecting the prostate. These two interventions may help reverse or better control prostate cancer cell activity and help bolster concurrent or future medical treatment.

Dr. Paolo Lissoni and his colleagues in Milan have been in the forefront of melatonin research as it applies to cancer prevention and treatment. In addition to work with breast cancer patients, they have administered melatonin in daily doses of 20 mg per day along with standard drugs and cancer treatments in cases of advanced lung, colon, and metastatic brain cancer. Their preliminary studies have shown that melatonin can improve outcomes in a significant number of cases; their research continues.

Melatonin Boosts Immune Function

There is considerable research evidence that melatonin boosts immune function; hence, the decline in melatonin levels as we age may be a significant contributing factor to the parallel decline in immune function. Receptors for melatonin have been found in lymphoid organs (such as the thymus gland and spleen) and on certain white blood cells. Some studies suggest that melatonin can help restore thymus gland function and prevent age-related thymus gland degeneration. In studies on mice, melatonin enhanced immune function even when the mice were given cortisol, a drug known to suppress the immune system. Melatonin supplementation also proved protective when the mice were subjected to various types of stress.

The research efforts of Drs. G.J. Maestroni and A. Contri and their colleagues have provided us with a glimpse into the workings of melatonin on the immune system. They have shown that the system's T-helper cells have receptors for melatonin and once stimulated by melatonin these immune cells provide a higher level of protection against infection and cancer development

Other investigations by Dr. Maestoni and Dr. Lissoni have shown that melatonin supplementation can produce a number of favorable benefits in HIV and AIDS patients when administered in conjunction with standard HIV drugs. Their studies provide definitive evidence that melatonin enhances immune function, even in individuals with very serious immune system diseases.

Melatonin and Alzheimer's Disease and Age-Related Cognitive Impairment

As an antioxidant, melatonin is unique in that it is both water- and fat-soluble. This means that it can intercept and suppress dangerous free radicals in every part of every cell in the body.

Melatonin may be the brain's most powerful antioxidant against free radical damage to its cells, damage that can contribute to the development of Alzheimer's disease and age-related cognitive dysfunction and can lead to neurodegenerative diseases such as multiple sclerosis, Parkinson's disease, and Lou Gehrig's disease.

In their quest to identify which elderly individuals are most at risk for memory loss or Alzheimer's disease, Italian gerontologists discovered that older individuals with higher melatonin levels showed better mental acuity than those with low levels. Japanese researchers made a similar finding, in that healthy functioning elderly subjects were shown to produce twice as much melatonin as Alzheimer's disease patients of like age.

Thus far, it's been established that melatonin can block some of the processes in the development of Alzheimer's disease in animals. The results of a landmark study published in the

December 11, 2001 issue of *Biochemistry* showed that in experiments with animals and human brain cell cultures, melatonin inhibited the formation of the amyloid protein that is the hallmark of Alzheimer's disease.

More research is required before any definitive statements can be made about melatonin and the prevention of Alzheimer's disease; however, it appears that the risk of excessive damage to our brain cells by oxygen free radicals may be another reason to consider the use of melatonin supplementation after age 40.

Dosage Ranges for Melatonin

For anti-aging, breast and prostate cancer prevention, an immune-system boost, or improved sleep quality, a night-time dosage of 200 mcg (.2 mg) to 3,000 mcg (3 mg) is typically used. This range may seem a large one, but individuals will respond differently. It's best to start with a small dose, in the range of 200 to 300 mcg, and work up, based on results. Doses that are too high can produce vivid dreams that may waken you in the night, morning grogginess, headaches, or abdominal cramps.

Always take melatonin at night, to correspond with the body's natural melatonin release cycle and to optimize its benefits: sleep quality will be enhanced, the immune system will be strengthened, and there will be sufficient clearance time to avoid any morning drowsiness.

Therapeutic doses as an adjunct to the treatment of a particular disease or condition, often in the range of 5 to 75 mg per day, should be undertaken only with the knowledge of a physician who is able to monitor blood levels and other parameters. These applications and dosages are still experimental; their long-term safety is unknown. However, melatonin testing in humans and animals indicates that it is nontoxic.

Contraindications and Drug-Nutrient Interactions

Some cases of depression can be aggravated by melatonin supplementation. A few antidepressant drugs stimulate the production of melatonin, while others, such as fluoxetine (Prozac), may lower melatonin levels. The prudent course is not to combine melatonin with any drug that targets brain chemistry or neurotransmitter levels (such as antidepressants or drugs designed to manage bipolar disease, schizophrenia, and related conditions).

10. Growth Hormone: A New and Promising Intervention

Growth hormone is a protein hormone (not a steroid) that is produced and secreted by the pituitary gland in the brain. Like estrogen, progesterone, testosterone, and melatonin, growth hormone secretions and blood levels decline as we age. The daily release of growth hormone averages about 500 mcg at age 20, then falls to 200 mcg at 40 and to 25 mcg by age 80. This drop in growth hormone secretion directly affects the release of Insulin-like Growth Factor-I (IGF-1) from the liver, the hormone-like substance that elicits powerful anti-aging effects on most body tissues. Because IGF-1 will be secreted only when influenced by growth hormone, lower blood levels of growth hormone mean lower levels of IGF-1.

A startling recent discovery is that the pituitary gland itself is not responsible for this fall-off in growth hormone secretion and blood level. It will continue to produce abundant amounts well into our 70s and 80s—unlike estrogen, progesterone, or testosterone whose actual synthesis declines with age. Growth hormone levels in the blood are affected by a decline in the hormone that stimulates its release, the so-called growth hormone releasing factors (GHRH) that are secreted by the hypothalamus gland, which sits above the pituitary gland in the brain.

Most of the release of growth hormone occurs in bursts at night during slow wave sleep, with the remainder secreted in smaller bursts during the day. Exercise, especially intensive weight training, and a low glycemic diet will enhance growth hormone secretion. (The secretions are suppressed when insulin levels are high.). Ultimately, the liver secretes less IGF-1, all of which results in an acceleration of the aging process.

Reversing the Aging Process with Growth Hormone

Growth hormone replacement or supplementation with natural agents that stimulate the release of growth hormone have reversed signs of aging in both human and animal studies. By returning IGF-1 blood levels to more youthful levels, subjects have experienced a multitude of anti-aging benefits, among them

- improved immune function;
- increased sexual potency and function;
- increased muscle strength, muscle mass and energy;
- decreased body fat;
- elevated mood;
- improved sleep patterns;
- improved memory;
- improved skin thickness, texture, and reduced wrinkle lines;
- restoration of hair color;
- improved vision.

The most pronounced of these effects have been observed in patients whose IGF-1 blood levels are at 350 ng/ml or greater, a level which some anti-aging doctors claim can reverse these features of aging by up to 20 years in older subjects. Blood levels in this range can be achieved only by regular injections of growth hormone administered by a physician who is trained in anti-aging medicine. Experimental data shows that growth hormone replacement not only enhances immune function to a marked degree, but it can regenerate the thymus gland, which is typically quite shriveled by age 40 and is almost undetectable by age 60.

Growth hormone injections are expensive, however, and have been known to cause side effects, especially in subjects where IGF-1 levels approached 400 ng/ml. The most common include swelling of the feet, fluid retention, joint pains, carpal tunnel syndrome and, more rarely, allergic responses. Because they are a relatively new intervention, their long-term safety has not been established.

Boosting IGF-1 blood levels above 290-300 ng/ml is cause for concern, in my view, as a number of research papers have correlated higher IGF-1 levels with an increased risk of breast and prostate cancer. We do know that IGF-1 increases the replication rate of certain cells in the body by virtue of its anabolic properties. There is evidence that individuals who have received growth hormone injections during their lifetimes to address a deficiency that would otherwise result in dwarfism or growth failure experience slightly higher rates of certain cancers than those who were not given injections to address the same conditions. For these reasons, patients with a previous history of cancer are advised against growth hormone injections, although to this point, older subjects receiving growth hormone injections for anti-aging purposes have not exhibited increased incidences of any type of cancer according to the published data.

Some evidence suggests that growth hormone replacement may actually help prevent cancer due to its rejuvenating effect on the immune system. In his book, *Grow Young with HGH*, Ronald Klatz reports a case of a significant drop in a patient's prostate specific antigen (PSA) level following growth hormone injections. The patient had a very high initial PSA level, between 50 and 60, and a needle biopsy confirmed adenocarcinoma in the prostate gland. He refused surgery and instead was treated with growth hormone injections, along with melatonin and DHEA supplementation. The patient's PSA level subsequently fell back within the normal range.

More research must be undertaken on growth hormone injections and cancer risk before we will know for certain whether the blood levels of IGF-1 achieved by this method are entirely safe for everyone. In the meantime, many anti-aging experts favor natural ingestible supplements as an alternative to injections.

Growth Hormone Secretagogues

A combination of certain amino acids, taken orally at specific dosages, can stimulate the pituitary gland to release greater quantities of growth hormone and elevate IGF-1 blood levels to match those we experienced in our mid-thirties. Studies show that supplementation with these amino acid combinations, collectively known as a growth hormone secretagogue (pronounced se-kre-ta-gog) can raise IGF-1 blood levels to 275 ng/ml, which may be safer than the 350 to 400 ng/ml that occur with growth hormone injections.

In one three-month study with a proven growth hormone secretagagogue supplement, blood levels of IGF-1 increased by 30 percent on average over a twelve-week period. Thirty-six participants, men and women over the age of 40, reported a range of effects in self-assessment scores, including:

- improvement in muscular strength: reported by 58 percent of participants
- increase in muscle size: 42 percent
- body fat reduction: 68 percent
- increase in energy: 74 percent
- improvements in skin texture: 47 percent

- improved skin thickness: 32 percent
- reduction in wrinkles (disappearance or reversal): 37 percent
- improvement in general healing capacity: 21 percent
- improvement in joint and back flexibility: 37 percent
- felt their immune system was stronger: 47 percent
- improved sexual potency: 32 percent
- better sexual stamina (penile erection): 44 percent
- less frequent nighttime urination (in men): 66 percent
- improved mental energy and clarity: 53 percent
- improved attitude and mood elevation: 37 percent
- improvement in memory: 47 percent

In male subjects there was a reduction in PSA blood levels, which signifies that this intervention did not trigger prostate malignancy or enlargement. As well, blood sugar levels in diabetic subjects were shown to normalize and there was an improvement in both cardiac and pulmonary function during the course of the three-month trial. The author of the study, Dr D.M. Ladley, also noted that blood pressure was better controlled and an improvement in menopausal symptoms among affected women was seen in this test group.

Ladley, an authority on the use of growth hormone secretagogues, stated that improved energy, endurance, muscle mass and strength, and reduced body fat were among the most frequently reported benefits in the first four weeks of supplementation. New hair growth, restoration of hair color, thickening of the skin, and the disappearance of skin discoloration generally occurred between the eighth and the twelfth weeks, with continued improvement beyond the twelve-week term. There were no side effects reported from the use of growth hormone secretagogues by any of the participants in this study. They are generally well tolerated and no consistent incidences of adverse side effects have been reported.

Raising IGF-1 Blood Levels with Growth Hormone Secretagogues

The extent to which IGF-1 blood levels can be raised with the use of a growth hormone secretagagogue supplement depends largely on initial IGF-1 blood levels. In the study by Ladley, pre-supplementation measures ranged from 21 to 276 ng/ml. Those with the lowest values experienced the greatest increases in IGF-1 blood levels.

As a rule, growth hormone secretagogue supplementation cannot elevate blood levels of IGF-1 beyond 275 ng/ml. So before beginning a supplementation program, have your blood levels of IGF-1 evaluated by your physician. (The cost of this test is not usually covered by universal health care or private insurance plans.) If you are over 40 years of age and your current blood levels of IGF-1 are below 275 ng/ml, then it is likely you will see positive results if you add a growth hormone secretagogue to your overall anti-aging wellness program. I recommend that you have your IGF-1 blood levels re-evaluated after twelve weeks to note the level of change. If your blood levels are already above 275 ng/ml, then it is unlikely that you will see dramatic reversals in your body's signs of aging by taking this supplement, although some experts claim that anti-aging benefits still occur.

How to Choose and Use a Growth Hormone Secretagogue Supplement

The growth hormone business is rife with unproven, ineffective, or bogus products that are not worth your time or money. However, the most respected anti-aging medical professionals in the field frequently recommend a growth hormone secretagogue supplement formula to their patients and colleagues that is available under two trade names: PRO hGH Symbiotropin and Meditropin. With either, you drop two of the effervescent tablets into a glass of water before bedtime, allowing them to dissolve fully before drinking it down.

They are best taken on an empty stomach to eliminate the risk of other amino acids competing for entry into the brain at the same time, so it's advisable not to eat anything for a couple hours before retiring. The supplement is used for five consecutive days, followed by two days with no supplementation; then the cycle repeats. For simplicity, many people take this supplement Monday to Friday, skip Saturday and Sunday, and begin again on Monday.

Experts suggest that if your initial IGF-1 blood level is below 100 ng/ml, you should double the dosage (four tablets dissolved in water before bedtime) until your levels reach at least 200 ng/ml, at which point you can assume the normal dosage of two tablets per day. If you do not see a change in your blood levels of IGF-1 after ingesting two tablets a day for three months and your levels are below 275 ng/ml, then experts advise that you may be one of the rare cases where a doubling of the dosage is justified.

To me, the use of growth hormone secretagogues represents a breakthrough in anti-aging research. Thus far, only a few well-designed trials have been published or presented at major conferences that demonstrate their benefits, but these preliminary studies have been most impressive and many physicians trained in anti-aging medicine regularly recommend these supplements to patients over the age of 40. Investigations in the next few years should provide more definitive evidence of their ability to counter the aging process and are likely to better identify any adverse side effects that may result from their use.

Conclusion: When to Incorporate Anti-Aging Supplements into Your Program

Based on the available research, I believe that after age 40 your body requires additional supplements to slow, and in some instances reverse, the signs of aging and to increase your protection against cancer, heart disease, dementia, infections, sexual dysfunction, and a host of other age-related problems. I have outlined what I consider to be the most scientifically sound anti-aging supplement formulations. The following chart provides a rough timetable for the introduction of each. Some may be initiated sooner; refer to Step 7 for the appropriate age ranges.

Women—Age	Anti-Aging Supplements to Add
40	• CoQ10 with hawthorn
	• Immune and detoxification formula
45	• Glucosamine sulfate with anti-inflammatory herbs • Vitamin D and calcium • Growth hormone secretagogue (optional)
50	• Menopausal herbal formula • Melatonin (optional) • Libido enhancer (optional)
55	• Brain support formula
Men—Age	Anti-Aging Supplements to Add
40	• CoQ10 and hawthorn • Immune and detoxification formula • Prostate support nutrients
45	• Glucosamine sulfate and anti-inflammatory herbs • Growth hormone secretagogue (optional)
50	• Vitamin D and calcium • Libido enhancer (optional) • Melatonin (optional)
55	• Brain support formula

*For access to the references to Step 5 and additional education on wellness please visit the author's web site at **www.renaisante.com***

STEP 6

Set Your Health, Fitness and Anti-Aging Goals

You have absorbed a lot of information in Steps 1 through 5 about how to eat, exercise, and supplement your diet as part of a lifelong health and anti-aging program. The next step is to make that program work for you—to tailor its principles to your personal tastes, your busy schedule, your particular health concerns and specific goals.

The working tool that will help you design that custom program—and stick to it—is the Goal-Setting Wellness Planner. With the Planner, you will identify your objectives for overall health and desired body shape and anticipate those obstacles that might stand in your way or pull you off target. You will establish effective strategies to overcome the roadblocks and achieve your goals. And you will translate what you dream of accomplishing into a tangible and realistic plan for success.

In addition, the Planner can help you connect to the positive changes that will come when you adhere to the strategies you set for yourself. Savoring the rewards of a healthier lifestyle and a fit and age-resistant body and mind can keep you focused and motivated, equipped to resist the temptations that will inevitably pop up along the way.

When you write down your goals and specify your strategies, you greatly improve your chances of success. Don't skip over this step: it's vital to making the program work for you. So get a pen and put your commitment on record.

The Goal-Setting Wellness Planner

Weight goal

Record your current weight, then the weight range that you believe to be realistic and healthy for you. A five-pound difference should separate the upper and lower limits of the range that is your goal.

Current weight: _____

Upper weight limit goal: _____

Lower weight limit goal: _____

If you are setting out to lose weight, then establish the date by which you will reach your goal. Assume that you can lose one to two pounds a week, on average.

I confidently expect to achieve my weight goal by: _____

_____

_____

If you are attempting to gain weight through weightlifting, follow a healthy diet and include approximately 1.5 grams of protein each day for every one kilogram (2.2 pounds) you weigh. If you work hard, you can expect an average gain of 0.5 to one pound of muscle per month.

Body Shape

I am committed to maintaining a waistline measurement of:

_____

_____

Dress size [for women]: _____ I am committed to attaining a dress size of: _____

_____

I confidently expect to achieve this goal by: _____

_____

Exercise Program

Aerobic Fitness

The Step 3 fitness program of gentle endurance or aerobic activity to which I am committed is: _____

_____

Endurance exercise type (treadmill, jogging, stationary bike, etc.):

_____

_____

Exercise time or distance (per session): _____

_____

_____

Exercise frequency (times per week): _____

_____

_____

Resistance-Training Program

If you are at a level at which strength training is appropriate, write down your program.

Name of station or exercise	Number of sets	Number of reps per set

For split routine, my Day Two program is:

Name of station or exercise	Number of sets	Number of reps per set

The number of weight-training sessions that I plan to do each week is: _____

Alternate Resistance-Training Program (e.g. yoga, Pilates, boxercise, etc.)

Type: _____

_____

Number of sessions per week: _____

_____

Type: _____

_____

Number of Sessions per week: _____

_____

Dietary Strategies

Meat: The high-fat meat products I currently eat are:_____

_____

_____

_____

Solution: The low-fat flesh protein foods that I will eat instead because they make sense for me are: _____

_____

_____

Dairy: The high-fat dairy products that I currently eat are: _____

_____

_____

Solution: The low-fat dairy protein foods that I will eat instead because they make sense for me are: _____

_____

_____

Pastries: The high-fat pastries, cakes, doughnuts, and chocolate products that I eat are: _____

_____

_____

Solution: The lower-fat solution-substitution foods that I will eat instead are: _____

_____

Fried foods: The fried and chippy-dippy foods that I eat are: _____

_____

_____

Solution: The lower-fat alternatives to these fried foods that I will substitute are:_____

_____

_____

Frozen desserts and treats: The high-fat ice cream and related frozen desserts that I eat are:_____

_____

_____

Solution: The lower-fat alternatives to these high-fat desserts and treats that I will substitute are:_____

_____

_____

Chocolate bars: The chocolate bars and other high-fat chocolate products that I tend to eat are: _____

_____

_____

Solution: The low-fat alternatives I will substitute for chocolate bars and related high-fat chocolate products are: _____

_____

_____

Sugary beverages: The sugary beverages that add unnecessary calories to my diet are:_____

_____

_____

Solution: The no-calorie beverages and diluted juices that I will drink instead include: _____

_____

_____

Candy: The sugary candy products I eat too often are:

_____

_____

Solution: The no-calorie or lower-calorie solutions that will help me achieve my goal are: _____

_____

_____

Added sugar: The items in my diet that include too much added sugar are: _____

_____

Solution: My solution to reducing these added sugars in my diet is: _____

_____

Under the following complex-carbohydrate headings, list the foods you plan to increase in your daily life because of their health-promoting properties.

Fruits: _____

_____

Green leafy vegetables: _____

_____

_____

Cruciferous vegetables: _____

_____

_____

Orange-yellow and red vegetables: _____

_____

High-fiber grains and starchy carbohydrates: _____

_____

_____

High-fiber breakfast cereals: _____

_____

_____

High-fiber bread products: _____

_____

_____

Other High-fiber grains and noodles: _____

_____

_____

Peas and beans: _____

_____

Healthy soups: _____

_____

Caffeine: I will limit my intake of coffee and tea to _____ cups per day.

Alcohol: I will limit my intake of alcohol to _____ drinks per week.

Supplementation

The daily lifelong and anti-aging supplements I intend to ingest each day include:

1 _____

2 _____

3 _____

4 _____

5 _____

6 _____

7 _____

8 _____

9 _____

10 _____

Fiber Supplement

In addition to choosing higher-fiber foods, I will include a fiber supplement each day.

Yes _____ No _____

If yes, my strategy is: _____

_____

_____

_____

_____

_____

Rewards

The health strategies described in my Goal-Setting Wellness Planner are designed to achieve a positive outcome for my body and to enhance my quality of life. I will be rewarded on three levels: my general health and wellbeing, my appearance and body shape, and my self-esteem and self-image.

The specific benefits of succeeding with this program for me are these:

Health benefits (the disease-prevention results that are most important to me):_____

_____

_____

_____

_____

_____

Physical appearance (the changes to my body that I am most eager to see):_____

_____

_____

Psychological benefits (how my fitter, healthier, leaner body will affect my life): _____

_____

_____

_____

Self-image:_____

_____

_____

_____

Social life: _____

_____

_____

_____

Willingness to participate in new activities:_____

_____

_____

_____

I am deeply committed to implementing these changes to experience and enjoy the rewards they will bring to my life.

_____   _____

Signature   Date

The Power of a Contract

Congratulations! You have just entered a new realm of commitment and opportunity. The simple act of writing out your goals and intentions has initiated a powerful shift from simply wishing for something to happen, to signing a contract with yourself to make it happen. It's the moment in which you can confidently declare: This is what I stand for now; this is what I am committed to achieving for myself and for my life.

And you have a concrete plan for incorporating the principles of my program into your everyday routine. You can see, realistically, how your plan will fit in with the other elements of your life. In the end, your wellness goals must become an integral part of your lifestyle; with the Goal-Setting Wellness Planner you have taken the first step towards that objective.

*For access to the references to Step 6 and additional education on wellness please visit the author's web site at **www.renaisante.com***

STEP 7

Stay on Track

One of the greatest challenges of any lifestyle change is being motivated tomorrow to achieve the goals of today. There's no escaping the fact that if you really want to reach your objectives, you have to work at them over the long haul. As the trite but true saying goes, "Success is 10 percent inspiration and 90 percent perspiration."

There is an energizing rush that accompanies the decision to accomplish a big goal; a fresh beginning is always exciting. But how many times have you started out of the blocks with a burst of enthusiasm only to find that your zest for the finish line soon slips away? It's easy to understand how it happens, given the myriad demands and choices of day-to-day living. You are pulled in so many directions by work, family, and social obligations that finding the time and energy to maintain an additional commitment to personal wellness can be difficult.

Expect your old habits to put up a strong fight too, luring you back to familiar comfort zones at the first sign of stress or fatigue. Watching television requires less effort than walking or jogging. The grocery stores are filled with your favorite high-fat foods, all enticingly displayed. There is a fast-food restaurant or doughnut shop at almost every urban intersection in North America. To resist these temptations, you need a strategy for staying on track until the necessary changes in your lifestyle become comfortable and habitual.

I urge you to adopt a few simple routines that will build one day's dedication on the next until you reach the goals you have set for yourself. By performing two specific tasks every day and two others every week you will keep your level of commitment high.

The Two Daily Steps

1. Every morning for the first 30 days, review your Goal Setting and Wellness Planner to re-ignite your dedication to success.

   This easy ritual will prepare you for the day's activities, allow you to anticipate the obstacles that may arise, and remind you of the priority of your health-related intentions. It takes only a minute or two and can make the difference between accomplishing your goals and losing ground to former bad habits.

2. Every evening, fill out the Daily Food, Fiber, and Exercise Journal (Appendix 2) to monitor your progress.

   To ensure you are following your personal nutritional and exercise program, keep a record of your performance, at least until its guidelines are internalized and automatic. At the end of each day, use the journal to record the foods and beverages you've consumed, the supplements taken, and the exercise program completed. Remember that your ideal daily nutritional components comprise:

   - one low-fat dairy protein meal,
   - two low-fat flesh protein meals,
   - 8 to 15 fiber points,
   - a maximum of two servings of olive or peanut oil,
   - 6 to 8 glasses of water,
   - at least four carbohydrate foods per day that are loaded with disease-protective nutrients.

You will find that the ritual of reporting to yourself, on paper, will often stop you in your tracks when you are tempted to cheat in moments of weakness; similarly, it will strengthen your commitment to your exercise program. My experiences with hundreds of nutrition clients and the published research of others prove that this self-monitoring tool is one of the most effective ways to maintain the program, especially in the early stages. The simple truth is that people who keep daily food and exercise records when they are trying to change their lifestyle habits perform much better in the long term than those who don't.

The Two Weekly Steps

1. Schedule your workout time in advance.

   Working exercise time into an already busy timetable is a tall order for most people. The only way to do it is to schedule your sessions in advance, before the calendar fills up completely. At the start of every week, take a look at the activities planned for the next seven days—work and family commitments, social functions, haircuts, doctors' appointments, anything that must be scheduled. With a clear picture of the week ahead, decide on which days and at what times you will to exercise— preferably for some period of time every day—and enter those times on your agenda. (If you plan for every day, you will succeed at least four or five days of the week, and that is not bad. If you plan for only three days, you will likely succeed only twice a week—not enough to reach your goals.)

   You may find yourself juggling occasionally in the middle of the week, but continue to write down those exercise times and schedule them like any other important appointment you have to keep. To decide that you can't find the time to exercise probably means that you haven't acknowledged it as a high priority. Exercise is a fundamental requirement of a healthy body. You cannot change that truth because you don't like it or because other distractions seem to fill up your days.

I've noticed that those who are willing to get up a little earlier in the morning to do their workout tend to have the best overall compliance. If you leave exercise until later in the day, some obligation may arise unexpectedly and you'll end up taking care of what seems urgent in the moment rather than what is essential in the long run. However, not everyone is a morning person, and body rhythm can dictate your best time. I prefer to exercise at the end of the workday. It helps me wind down, clears my head and refreshes me for the evening ahead. Whatever your timing, you'll soon find your workout so rejuvenating that you'll look forward to it; without it, you'll feel sluggish and out of sorts. Finding time for exercise will be a pleasure, not a challenge.

2. Make a weekly grocery list that is consistent with the program.

To ensure that you surround yourself with healthy foods, follow a shopping list that restocks your kitchen with the foods discussed in the program. Don't buy the foods that can sabotage your efforts. Baking desserts for family and friends is a common practice, but is feeding them the high-fat and sugar-sweetened treats that promote heart disease, diabetes, and other degenerative diseases a truly considerate gift? A better way to express your love is by preparing healthy alternatives to potentially harmful foods.

If you follow these strategies for staying on track—two steps every day and two steps every week—I guarantee that your performance and compliance will improve. With time, experience, and repetition you will eventually experience a breakthrough and within the first three months see the benefits of your efforts. Your clothes will start to fit better. You will have more energy. You'll feel toned and generally healthier. Even your taste buds will be transformed as you begin to savor wiser food choices. If you stay the course, the day will come when your body develops a healthy addiction to the positive feelings of wellbeing that result from regular exercise, supplementation, and a healthy diet.

Tracking Your Monthly Progress

As a means of measuring your longer-term progress, especially if weight loss or body shape change is among your goals, I advise you to complete a Monthly Body Shape Assessment (Appendix 4). The Assessment is a useful yardstick for tracking changes to your body's dimensions over time. Recording your waist, hip, chest, bicep, thigh, and calf measurements will confirm your changing contours, over and above any weight changes you may experience, and bolster your resolve to continue. Note your starting measurements today as a baseline and make extra copies of the form if you wish to continue tracking for more than a year.

Other Important Resources

In addition to these strategies for staying on track, there are a number of highly effective resources that I have found invaluable in my own life and in working with patients.

- Health Magazines

  Converts to the wellness lifestyle want to stay up to date with the scientific research relating to health, and I have found that those who continue to educate themselves on the subject remain more connected to the principles of healthy living. There are many excellent magazines designed for the general consumer that inform and entertain in everyday language. I especially recommend the following, but check out a well-stocked magazine stand or your local library for the broadest selection.

Longevity	*Men's Health*
In-Health	*Health*
Shape	*Runner's World*

Find one or two that appeal to you and subscribe. Their arrival at your door every month will reinforce your interest and your commitment.

- CDs, DVDs, Audio and Video Tapes

  The market is flooded with multimedia items aimed at health, nutrition, and fitness interests. Just like magazines, they can provide the incentive to stick with your program. If you don't want to join a club or can't always get out, a DVD or video program of aerobic fitness, Pilates or power yoga can provide the convenience of a workout at home.

- Pictures

  If it's true that a picture is worth a thousand words, find a photo of your trim and fit ideal in a magazine or newspaper. Post it where you'll see it at least twice a day—on your mirror, at your desk, over the sink, or on that perennial notice board, the refrigerator door. Remember, your goals have to be realistic, so choose a model that is within your reach. Or find a photo of yourself at your peak of physical fitness, possibly an even more effective incentive because it's proof that you can succeed.

- Inspirational Quotes

  Quotations and sayings can have the same positive effects as photographs, creating productive and playful reinforcement.

Watch for expressions that are meaningful to you and display them prominently. Here are a few of my favourites:

"If it is to be, it's up to me."

"Whoever wants to reach a distant goal must take many small steps." (Helmut Schmidt)

"I never knew a man worth his salt who, in the long run, deep down in his heart, did not appreciate the grind and discipline necessary to become a champion." (Vince Lombardi)

- Sufficient Rest

Breaking out of a rut requires energy. The extra energy needed for this program may leave you fatigued in the early stages and if you are tired, you'll lose your enthusiasm. Fight those feelings either by going to bed half an hour earlier than usual or catching a power nap sometime during the day. You'll be delighted at how much easier it is to maintain the regimen if you feel adequately refreshed and energized.

- Positive People

Thousands of people have joined the wellness movement since the early 1970s. These high-energy individuals can be a tremendous source of inspiration if you get close enough for the effects to rub off. You do not need to copy their exact lifestyles or fitness routines, but simply allow their positive attitudes to recharge your psychological batteries. Joining a fitness club, preferably one that is close enough to encourage regular use, can put you in contact with like-minded men and wo-men of almost every age. Sign up for an aerobics class, an aqua-fit course, or a seniors' fitness session. Get to know your fellow participants and surround yourself with those who will help you succeed.

Remember that attitudes are contagious. Not everyone shares the same philosophy; some people are content to smoke two packs a day, eat junk food, and pay no heed to preventive health. Those who boldly proclaim that they are here for a good time rather than a long time may change their minds after suffering their first heart attacks or bouts of cancer. Ultimately, you know what is in your own best interest. Don't let others deflate your enthusiasm for wellness and the benefits it will bring to your life.

• *The Meschino Optimal Living Program*—Again

This book is chock-full of health, fitness, and anti-aging information. It's unlikely you will remember all of it the first time through. One of the best ways to stay on track is to read it three or four times from cover to cover, or scan the sections that you highlighted during your initial read. With every revisit, new information will jump off the page and new ideas will be triggered in your mind.

On Your Way

I hope you have enjoyed and learned from this book. My objective in writing it was to provide you with a clear understanding of how nutrition, exercise, and supplementation work together to improve your physical and mental health, to prevent degenerative illnesses, and to slow or reverse the aging process. Its principles have been developed over many years and relayed to thousands of people through seminars, audio and video tapes, individual and group counseling sessions, and in the health and anti-aging magazine columns I have written. *The Meschino Optimal Living Program* draws together all the elements in one comprehensive program.

It is my hope that you will put these strategies to work for you. Not only will you be happier with the way you look and feel, but you'll be rewarded with the buoyant quality of life that only a fit, lean, well-functioning, and, dare I say, sexier body can provide. Many of us are living proof that you can regain and maintain a vibrant body, long after your peers have succumbed to joint and muscle decay, runaway weight gain and obesity, adult onset diabetes, high blood pressure, angina, prostate enlargement, or other age-related conditions. Regardless of your starting point, you can choose a different path.

I congratulate you on investing the time to discover the principles of this program and its scientific rationale. I wish you the best of success in the pursuit of your objectives and I conclude by encouraging you to eat smart, live well, and take control of your physical wellbeing—today and for life.

*For access to the references to Step 7 and additional education on wellness please visit the author's web site at **www.renaisante.com***

Appendix I

The Fiber Scoreboard

Here is a practical and reliable method of determining your daily fiber intake. You should accumulate eight to 15 fiber points a day to meet the recommendations of the cancer and heart associations and other leading authorities. For any food not listed here, divide the number of grams of fiber shown on the label by three to determine the number of fiber points in a serving size.

Cereal Products

	Portion Size	Calories	Fiber Points
Kellogg's All Bran	$^1/_2$ cup	90	3.5
Kellogg's Bran Buds	$^1/_2$ cup	90	3.5
Cooked buckwheat groats (kasha)	1 cup	160	3.0
Cooked bulgur	1 cup	160	3.0
Nabisco 100% Bran	$^1/_2$ cup	105	3.0
Cooked oatmeal	$^3/_4$ cup	212	2.5
Quaker Corn Bran	$^2/_3$ cup	115	2.0
Kellogg's Bran Flakes - plain	1 cup	90	1.5
- with raisins	1 cup	110	2.0
Most	1 cup	200	2.5
Kellogg's Bran Chex	$^2/_3$ cup	90	1.5
Fruitful Bran	$^3/_4$ cup	110	1.5
Shredded Wheat - large biscuit	1	74	0.75
- spoon size	1 cup	168	1.5
General Foods' Grape Nuts	$^1/_4$ cup	105	1.0
Health Valley Sprouts (7 with raisins)	$^1/_4$ cup	105	1.5
Kellogg's 40% Bran Flakes	$^3/_4$ cup	95	2.0

(continued)

Cereal Products (*Continued*)

	Portion Size	Calories	Fiber Points
Quaker Oats - Life	$^2/_3$ cup	110	1.0
Kellogg's Nutri-Grain	$^2/_3$ cup	110	1.0
Kellogg's Nutri-Grain Wheat	$^3/_4$ cup	105	1.0
Post 40% Bran Flakes	$^2/_3$ cup	95	2.0
Quaker 100% Natural Cereal	$^1/_4$ cup	110	1.0
Kellogg's Special K	1 cup	105	0.25
Kellogg's Total	1 cup	115	1.0
Purina Wheat Chex	$^2/_3$ cup	105	1.0
Wheaties	1 cup	115	1.0
Kellogg's Corn Flakes	$^3/_4$ cup	70	1.0
Kellogg's Cracklin' Oat Bran	$^1/_2$ cup	110	1.0
Kellogg's Fruit N' Fiber	$^1/_2$ cup	90	1.0
Puffed Wheat	1 cup	43	1.0
Kellogg's Raisin Bran	$^1/_2$ cup	95	1.0
Cooked wheat	$^2/_3$ cup	101	0.75
Honey Nut Cheerios	$^3/_4$ cup	115	0.5
Honey Nut Crunch Raisin Bran	$^1/_2$ cup	95	0.5
Kellogg's Corn Pops	1 cup	105	0.25
Purina Corn Chex	1 cup	115	0.25
Cheerios	$^1/_2$ cup	60	0.25
Post Toasties Corn Flakes	$^1/_2$ cup	60	0.5

Hot Cereal

	Portion Size	Calories	Fiber Points
Old Fashioned Quaker Oats	$^3/_4$ cup	110	1.0
Quick Quaker Oats	$^3/_4$ cup	110	1.0

Fruits

	Portion Size	Calories	Fiber Points
Apple (raw)	1 med.	70	1.0
	1 large	80-100	1.5
Applesauce	$^1/_2$ cup	115	0.5
Apricots (whole, raw)	1	17	0.5
Avocado	1 med.	306	1.0
Banana	1 med.	105	1.0
Blackberries	$^1/_2$ cup	27	1.5
Blueberries	1 cup	82	2.0
Boysenberries	1 cup	66	2.0
Cantaloupe	1 cup	57	0.5
Cherries	10	49	0.5
Cranberries (raw)	$^1/_4$ cup	12	0.5
Cranberry sauce	$^1/_2$ cup	246	1.0
Dates (pitted)	2	39	0.5
Figs (dried)	3	120	3.5
Figs (fresh)	1	30	0.5
Grapefruit (whole)	1	80	0.5
Grapes (white, red, or black)	15-20	70	0.5
Honeydew melon	3" slice	42	0.5
Kiwi	1 med.	46	0.5
Mango	1 med.	135	1.25
Nectarine	1 med.	67	1.0
Orange	1 med.	34	0.75
Papaya	1 med.	117	1.0
Passion fruit	1 med.	18	1.0
Peach - raw	1 med.	38	0.75
- canned in syrup	2 halves	70	0.5

(continued)

Fruits (*Continued*)

	Portion Size	Calories	Fiber Points
Pear	1 med.	98	1.5
Persimmon	1 med.	32	1.0
Pineapple - raw	¹/₂ cup	41	0.5
- canned	¹/₂ cup	60-75	0.5
Plums	1 med.	36	0.5
Pomegranate	1 med.	104	0.75
Prunes (pitted)	3	122	0.75
Raisins	1 tbsp.	29	0.5
	¹/₂ cup	192	1.25
Raspberries (raw, fresh, or frozen)	¹/₂ cup	20	1.5
Raspberry jam	1 tbsp.	75	0.5
Rhubarb (stewed)	1 cup	104	0.75
Strawberries (raw)	1 cup	45	1.0
Strawberry jam	1 tbsp.	90	0.5
Tangerine	1 med.	37	1.0
Watermelon	1 thick slice	68	0.5

Packaged/Prepared Fruits

	Portion Size	Calories	Fiber Points
Birds Eye frozen strawberries (in syrup)	¹/₂ cup	160	0.5
Del Monte Bartlett pear halves	¹/₂ cup	80	0.75
Del Monte fruit cocktail	¹/₂ cup	80	0.25
Del Monte pineapple chunks (own juice)	¹/₂ cup	70	0.5
Del Monte sliced pineapple			
Del Monte sliced pineapple (own juice)	¹/₂ cup	70	0.5
Del Monte yellow cling peach halves	¹/₂ cup	50	1.0

(continued)

Packaged/Prepared Fruits (*Continued*)

	Portion Size	Calories	Fiber Points
Dale sliced pineapple	$^1/_2$ cup	95	0.5
Dale sliced pineapple (own juice)	$^1/_2$ cup	70	0.5
Libby's fruit cocktail	$^1/_2$ cup	85	0.5
Libby's Lite yellow cling peaches (packed in fruit juice)	$^1/_2$ cup	50	0.5
Sun Sweet whole prunes	5-6	120	3.0

Vegetables

	Portion Size	Calories	Fiber Points
Artichoke - boiled	1 med.	53	1.0
- hearts	$^1/_2$ cup	37	0.75
Asparagus	$^1/_2$ cup	15	0.5
Avocado	1 med.	310	2.0
Bamboo shoots	$^1/_2$ cup	21	0.75
Beets	$^1/_2$ cup	33	1.0
Broccoli	$^1/_2$ cup	20	1.0
Broccoli spears	2	20	1.0
Brussels sprouts (cooked)	$^3/_4$ cup	36	1.0
Cabbage (raw or cooked)	$^1/_2$ cup	8	0.5
Carrots (raw)	$^1/_4$ cup	10	0.5
Carrot sticks	4-5	10	0.5
Carrots (cooked)	$^1/_2$ cup	20	0.5
Cauliflower (raw or cooked)	1 cup	16	1.0
Celery (hearts)	$^1/_4$ cup	5	0.5
Celery stalks	1	8	0.5
Chinese-style vegetables	$^1/_2$ cup	79	1.0

(*continued*)

Vegetables (*Continued*)

	Portion Size	Calories	Fiber Points
Corn - popcorn	4 cups	90	2.0
- corn on the cob	1 med.	70	1.5
- cooked or canned	$^1/_2$ cup	64	1.5
Cucumber (raw)	$^1/_2$ med.	8	0.5
Eggplant	2 slices	42	1.0
Endive (raw)	20 leaves	10	0.5
Greens, cooked: collards, beet greens, dandelion, kale, Swiss chard, turnip greens	$^1/_2$ cup	20	1.0
Lettuce (Boston, leaf, or iceberg)	1 cup	10	0.5
Mushrooms	5 small	14	0.5
	10 small	28	1.0
Okra (raw, cooked, or frozen)	$^1/_2$ cup	13	0.5
Onion	1 med.	65	0.75
Parsley (chopped)	4 tbsp.	4	0.5
Parsnip (cooked)	1 large	76	1.0
Peas and carrots (frozen)	$^1/_2$ pkg.	40	2.0
Peppers	$^1/_2$ cup	13	0.5
- dried crushed peppers	1 tsp.	7	0
Potatoes	1 small	95	1.0
Radishes	3	5	0.25
Rhubarb (cooked)	$^1/_2$ cup	100	1.0
Rutabaga	$^1/_2$ cup	40	1.0
Sauerkraut (canned)	$^2/_3$ cup	15	1.0
Spinach - raw	1 cup	8	1.0
- cooked	$^1/_2$ cup	26	2.5
Summer squash (boiled)	$^1/_2$ cup	14	0.75
- Winter squash (baked)	$^1/_2$ cup	63	1.0
Sweet potato (baked)	1 large	254	1.75

(continued)

Vegetables (*Continued*)

	Portion Size	Calories	Fiber Points
Tomatoes	1 small	22	0.5
	1/2 cup	22	0.5
Turnip - raw	1/4 cup	8	0.5
- cooked	1/2 cup	16	0.75
Watercress (raw)	1/2 cup	4	0.5
Yams (cooked or baked in skin)	1 med.	156	2.0
Zucchini (raw)	1/2 cup	11	0.75
Del Monte cream style			
golden sweet corn	1/2 cup	80	1.0
Del Monte Early Garden spinach	1/2 cup	25	2.0
Del Monte Early Garden sweet peas	1/2 cup	60	2.0
Del Monte whole green beans	1/2 cup	20	1.0

Canned Vegetables

	Portion Size	Calories	Fiber Points
Del Monte whole kernel			
Family Style corn	1/2 cup	70	1.0
Green Giant asparagus cuts	1/2 cup	20	1.0
Green Giant cream style corn	1/2 cup	100	1.0
Green Giant french style			
cut green beans	1/2 cup	18	1.0
Green Giant kitchen cut green beans	1/2 cup	20	1.0
Green Giant mushrooms	2 oz.	14	0.5
Green Giant sweet peas	1/2 cup	60	1.75
Green Giant whole kernel corn	1/2 cup	90	1.5
Le Sueur Early June peas	1/2 cup	60	2.0
Libby's Natural Pack mixed vegetables	1/2 cup	60	1.0
Veg-All	1/2 cup	35	1.0

Frozen Vegetables

	Portion Size	Calories	Fiber Points
Birds Eye broccoli spears	$^1/_2$ cup	25	1.0
Birds Eye cooked winter squash	$^1/_2$ cup	45	1.0
Birds Eye cut green beans	$^1/_2$ cup	25	1.0
Birds Eye green peas	$^1/_2$ cup	80	2.0
Birds Eye Italian Style vegetables	$^1/_2$ cup	110	1.0
Birds Eye Japanese Style vegetables	$^1/_2$ cup	100	1.0
Birds Eye Little Ears of Corn	2 ears	130	1.5
Birds Eye San Francisco Style vegetables	$^1/_2$ cup	100	0.75
Birds Eye sweet corn	$^1/_2$ cup	80	1.75
Seabrook Farms baby Brussels sprouts	$^1/_2$ cup	35	1.0

Legumes (Peas and Beans)

	Portion Size	Calories	Fiber Points
Black beans (cooked)	$^1/_2$ cup	100	3.0
Broad beans	$^3/_4$ cup	30	1.0
Northern navy beans	1 cup	160	5.0
Kidney beans	$^1/_2$ cup	150	3.0
Lima beans	$^1/_2$ cup	90	2.5
Pinto beans	$^1/_2$ cup	75	3.0
White beans dried before cooking	$^1/_2$ cup	160	5.0
- dried, canned, cooked	$^1/_2$ cup	80	2.5
Bean sprouts (raw)	$^1/_4$ cup	7	1.0
Chick-peas (garbanzo beans)			
- canned or cooked	$^1/_4$ cup	205	2.0
Chestnuts	3 large	29	1.0

(continued)

Legumes (Peas and Beans) (*Continued*)

	Portion Size	Calories	Fiber Points
Green (snap) beans (fresh or frozen)	¹/₂ cup	10	0.75
Lentils	¹/₂ cup	100	1.0
Peas (green, fresh or frozen)	¹/₂ cup	60	3.0
Black-eyed peas (frozen or canned)	¹/₂ cup	74	2.5
Split peas (dried or cooked)	¹/₂ cup	63	2.0

Breads

	Portion Size	Calories	Fiber Points
Bagel - plain	1	150	0.5
- whole wheat or pumpernickel	1	150	1.0
Boston brown bread	2 slices	100	1.0
Bread sticks	1	23	trace
Bulgur, dry	1 cup	548	4.5
Cornbread	1 piece	198	0.5
Cracked wheat bread	2 slices	120	1.0
Dark rye (whole grain) bread	2 slices	108	1.0
Dinner rolls	2	155	0.5
English muffins (whole wheat)	1	125	1.0
High-bran bread	2 slices	140	2.0
Pita - plain	1 large	240	0.5
- whole wheat	1 large	236	2.0
Pumpernickel	2 slices	116	1.0
Raisin bread	2 slices	140	0.75
Seven grain bread	2 slices	125	2.0
Sourdough bread	2 slices	136	0.5
White bread	2 slices	140	0.5

(continued)

Breads (*Continued*)

	Portion Size	Calories	Fiber Points
Whole wheat bread	2 slices	120	2.0
Whole wheat raisin bread	2 slices	140	2.0

Crackers

	Portion Size	Calories	Fiber Points
Fiber Med biscuits	1	152	3.3
Graham crackers	3	53	0.75
Ry-Krisps	3	64	0.5
Triscuits	2	50	0.75
Wheat Thins	6	58	0.75
Premium Saltine crackers	10	120	0.5
UNEEDA biscuits	6	130	0.5
Wasa Lite Rye Crispbread	3	90	1.0

Pasta

	Portion Size	Calories	Fiber Points
Macaroni			
- whole wheat, uncooked	$^1/_2$ cup	200	2.0
Spaghetti			
- whole wheat (uncooked)	$^1/_2$ cup	200	1.5
- plain (uncooked)	$^1/_2$ cup	200	1.0
- with tomato sauce	$^1/_2$ cup	220	2.0
Spinach noodles (uncooked)	$^1/_2$ cup	200	2.0
Spinach lasagna	1 serving	215	1.0
Tortellini with tomato sauce	1 cup	317	0.5

Rice

	Portion Size	Calories	Fiber Points
White (uncooked)	$^1/_2$ cup	79	0.75
Brown (uncooked)	$^1/_2$ cup	83	2.0
Instant rice	1 serving	79	0.25

Prepared Frozen Dinners (most are extremely high in salt)

	Portion Size	Calories	Fiber Points
Armour Chicken Burgundy Classic Lite Dinner	$11^1/_4$ oz.	240	2.0
Armour Chicken Fricassee Dinner Classic	$11^3/_4$ oz.	330	2.0
Armour Seafood Natural Herbs Classic Lite Dinner	$11^1/_2$ oz.	230	1.5
Armour Seafood Newburg Dinner Classic	$10^1/_2$ oz.	270	1.0
Armour Sliced Beef with Broccoli Classic Lite	$10^1/_4$ oz.	290	1.0
Norton Turkey Dinner	11 oz.	340	1.0
Swanson Hungry-Man Turkey Dinner	$18^1/_2$ oz.	630	2.0
Swanson Macaroni and Cheese Dinner	$12^1/_4$ oz.	380	2.0
Swanson Turkey Dinner	$11^1/_2$ oz.	340	2.0
Stouffer's Glazed Chicken with Vegetable Rice Lean Cuisine	$8^1/_2$ oz.	270	0.5
Stouffer's Spaghetti with Beef and Mushroom Sauce Lean Cuisine	$11^1/_2$ oz.	280	0.5

Soups

	Portion Size	Calories	Fiber Points
Campbell's Chunky Vegetable Soup	1 cup	104	1.0
Progresso Minestrone Soup	8 oz.	130	1.75
Progresso Green Split Pea Soup	1 cup	180	1.75
Potato soup	1 cup	178	2.75

Prepared Dinners

	Portion Size	Calories	Fiber Points
Ratatouille	$^1/_2$ cup	87	0.5
Mexican foods (low in fat; high in fiber)			
- Bean burrito (without cheese)	1 large	284	2.0
- Old El Paso Refried Beans	1 cup	200	4.0
Oriental Foods			
- Chicken and vegetable stir fry	1 cup	142	1.0
- Chop suey or chow mein	1 cup	85	0.75
- Chun King Chicken Chow Mein Pouch	6 oz.	90	1.0
- La Choy Fancy Chinese Mixed Vegetables (drained)	$^1/_2$ cup	12	1.0
- La Choy Shrimp Chow Mein	$^3/_4$ cup	60	0.5
- La Choy Sukiyaki	$^3/_4$ cup	70	1.0

(Data for the Fiber Scoreboard has been drawn from *The F-Plan Diet* by Audrey Eyton (Bantam Books, 1984), *The Food Book* by Bert Stern (Dell, 1987), the USDA Nutrient Data Research Group, and from my own research on brand food labeling.)

Appendix 2

The Daily Food, Fiber, and Exercise Journal

Food and Beverages   **Fiber Points**   Date: _____

Breakfast:

_____

_____   Type: _____

_____   Distance: _____

_____   Duration: _____

_____

Exercise

Lunch:

_____

_____   No: _____

_____   Yes: _____

_____

_____

Supplements:

Dinner:

_____

_____

_____

_____

_____

Snacks:

_____

_____

Total Fiber Points (goal is 8-15) _____

Make copies of the Daily Food, Fiber, and Exercise Journal form and use one every day to record your dietary intake and exercise participation. Here's an example.

The Daily Food, Fiber, and Exercise Journal: A Sample Entry

Food and Beverages   **Fiber Points**   **Date:** September 8

Breakfast:

Food	Fiber Points
½ cup All Bran cereal	3.5
8 oz. of skim milk	1
slice whole wheat toast with	1
whole fruit jam	0.5
green tea	

Exercise

Type: Power Walk

Distance: 3 Miles

Duration: 45 Mins

Lunch:

Food	Fiber Points
1 small tin water-packed salmon	
1 whole wheat bagel	1
1 cup fruit cocktail	1
low-salt soda water	

Supplements:

No: _____

Yes: √ _____

Dinner:

Food	Fiber Points
1 cup spaghetti with tomato sauce	4
1 white roll	0.5
mixed salad with olive oil & vinegar	1
diet soft drink	

Snacks:

Food	Fiber Points
4 cups low-fat popcorn	2

Total Fiber Points (goal is 8-15) _____ 14.5

Appendix 3

Food Preparation Guide

General Tips

- Non-stick pans allow you to cook without adding extra fat. If you have ordinary pans, use a non-stick spray instead of oiling or buttering them.
- Low-fat cooking doesn't have to be tasteless. Experiment with herbs and spices, adding them to soups, casseroles, pasta, salads, and popcorn.
- Use cooking methods that don't require added oil—try broiling, baking, microwaving, or steaming.
- Sauté in wine or broth instead of oil.

Low-Fat Flesh Protein Foods

- Broil, grill, or steam poultry and fish.
- Cook poultry and fish in a fondue, using consommé broth or a clear broth instead of oil.
- Poach poultry and fish in clear broth, vegetable juices, or water seasoned with lemon.
- Barbecue chicken or fish.
- Remove the skin from chicken, preferably before cooking it. Choose white rather than dark meat.
- The fish highest in omega 3 fats are salmon, mackerel, herring, trout, sardines, shad, anchovies, and albacore tuna. Clams, crab, and mussels also contain omega 3 fats.
- Add seafood, such as clams or mussels, to pasta dishes.

- Choose water-packed, not oil-packed, canned fish. Rinse the salt from canned fish.
- Mix tuna or salmon salad with low-fat yogurt or low-fat mayonnaise instead of regular mayonnaise.
- Frozen dinners that are labeled "light" or "low-calorie" are not necessarily low in fat. Read the label carefully and choose only those that have fewer than eight grams of fat per 300-calorie serving.

Low-Fat Dairy Protein

- Drink milk with no more than 1% M.F.
- Eat plain yogurt that contains 1% M.F. or less. Beware of yogurts sweetened with sugar that can add unwanted refined sugar calories to your diet. You can make your own flavors by adding fresh fruit and perhaps a dry high-fiber cereal for crunch and texture.
- Eat cheese with 3% M.F. or less. Most solid cheeses are more than 25% M.F. (Cheddar, for example, is 32% M.F., and brick is 29% M.F.)
- If you order pizza, ask that they use only half the regular amount of cheese or no cheese at all. Avoid high-fat toppings such as bacon, sausage, pepperoni, and olives. Even better, buy a pizza shell or plain frozen pizza and add your own vegetable toppings.
- Use buttermilk made from skim milk.
- Spread low-fat cheese thinly on bread as a substitute for butter or margarine.

Breakfast Cereals

- Choose cereals that are low in sugars and high in fiber. Refer to the Fiber Scoreboard (Appendix 1) for appropriate selections.

Bread

- Choose bread that is high in natural fiber but low in fat: whole wheat, pumpernickel, rye, whole wheat bagels, and pita.
- Toasting bread increases its fiber content.
- Don't butter your bread (butter is 80 percent fat) and try to avoid margarine.
- Whole fruit jam is a good alternative to butter or margarine. Read the label to be sure it is high in fruit and low in sugar.
- Spread low-fat cheese on your bread as part of a low-fat dairy meal.
- Avoid egg breads and bread products that are high in saturated fats.
- Try making yogurt "cheese" by taking low-fat yogurt and letting it drain through a fine sieve or a piece of cheese-cloth overnight.

Crackers and Biscuits

- Avoid crackers made with palm or coconut oil. Some healthy choices are rice crackers, bread sticks, melba toast, soda crackers, and matzoth.
- Avoid all fried biscuits, chips, nachos, and tortillas, regardless of the kind of oil used in their processing. Not only are they high in total fat, but the oil they were fried in may have been heated to high temperatures and left exposed to light and air, causing it to become carcinogenic.
- For snacks, try baked, crispy bread products, such as pita chips and bagel chips.
- Fiber cookies, often available at drug stores, make great snacks.

Fruit

- All kinds of fruit are good for you.
- The best cholesterol-lowering fruits are apples, peaches, pears, plums, nectarines, the white rind of citrus fruits, blueberries, strawberries, raspberries, mangoes, and papaya.
- Anti-cancer fruits are those with lots of vitamin C or beta-carotene. Citrus fruits and kiwis have the most vitamin C. Orange fruits, including cantaloupe, apricots, peaches, nectarines, oranges, mangoes, and watermelon are highest in beta-carotene.
- Fruit salad makes a wonderful dessert.

Vegetables

- Cruciferous vegetables—Brussels sprouts, cabbage, turnips, cauliflower, broccoli, bok choy and turnips—are excellent anti-cancer foods.
- Vegetables high in beta-carotene are also good anti-cancer foods. Carrots, squash, eggplant, and other orange/yellow vegetables, as well as broccoli, spinach, and dark green, leafy vegetables, are all high in beta-carotene.
- Try vegetables raw, steamed, broiled, microwaved, marinated, or stir-fried. Serve them with rice.
- Carrots, potatoes, and peas are high in cholesterol-cruncher fiber, especially good for your heart.
- Bake or boil potatoes. Instead of butter, use low-fat yogurt (1% M.F.) or ultra low-fat sour cream (up to 3% M.F.). Try baked potatoes without adding anything and give your taste buds a chance to explore.
- Avocados are high in monounsaturated fat (the same kind of fat found in olive and peanut oils). However, they are

also high in vitamins and minerals, so you may eat small amounts occasionally. Try two small slices in a sandwich along with tomatoes, cucumbers, and alfalfa sprouts. A little bit of avocado can be a good substitute for cheese and other animal-based foods.

- Salads are a healthy way to consume vegetables. Spinach salad, chef's salad, and mixed green salads, tossed with a light olive oil and vinegar dressing, are the best options. Shredded cabbage, seasoned with a light olive oil and vinegar dressing, is a tasty alternative to lettuce.

- Try flavored vinegars to add variety to your salads. You can purchase them or make your own by dropping fresh herbs or garlic into wine vinegar and letting the mixture sit for a week.

Grains

- Rice is best steamed or boiled.
- Brown rice is better than white rice because of its high fiber content.

Peas and Beans

- If you are using canned peas or beans, put them in a strainer and rinse with water to get rid of the excess salt and oil.

- If you are cooking dried beans yourself, cover them with cold water overnight. The next day, drain and cook in fresh water until they are tender. Many beans and peas are an excellent source of both cholesterol-cruncher and colon-cleaner fiber, contain less than 20 percent of their calories as fat, and provide additional protein and slow-release carbohydrates to the body (so they don't upset blood sugar). They should be included in your diet frequently.

Pasta

- All noodles are acceptable, but egg noodles are higher in cholesterol.
- Whole wheat noodles and spinach noodles are especially good choices.
- Gnocchi, made from potatoes and flour, are another good option. They are a good source of protein, low in fat, but high in carbohydrates.
- Use light (low-fat) tomato sauces. Sauté vegetables in water or olive oil before adding to the sauce. Green peppers, red peppers, mushrooms, onions, and zucchini are all excellent choices. Add clams, mussels, scallops, or chicken if you wish.
- Do not use cream sauces or meat sauces. They are very high in fat.
- Bottled tomato sauces with meat are also high in fat. Go to the refrigerator section of the grocery store and buy a fresh marinara sauce and add your own fresh vegetables. The vegetables will improve the taste, add vitamins, and dilute the fat content.

Oils

- Use olive oil for salad dressings or for sautéing vegetables. Canola oil is also acceptable.
- Use peanut oil for stir-frying.
- Vegetable oil sprays (such as Pam) are acceptable substitutes for vegetable oils.
- Use fat-free, butter-flavored sprinkles instead of butter, margarine, or oil.

Snack Foods and Desserts

- The urge to eat dessert is often a result of delayed satiety after the meal you have just eaten. It takes more than 30 minutes for your brain's appetite center to shut off. So wait for 10 to 15 minutes after a meal before deciding to indulge in a dessert. You will probably find that you are satisfied and no longer crave a treat.

- Get up from the table before dessert is served and go for a walk. This will curb your appetite and help you digest your meal.

- Unbuttered, low-fat popcorn is the best late night snack food. Popcorn made in an air popper has the least amount of fat. Use a microwave popcorn that contains no more than 1.2 grams of fat per three cups.

- Munchies such as potato chips, nacho chips, and cheesies are very high in fat.

- For healthy munchies, try melba toast with salsa, rice crackers, raisins, baked bagel slices, or low-fat biscuits.

- Make your own chips. Cut corn tortillas into pieces, lightly coat a baking dish with non-stick spray, and bake at 375 degrees (200C) until they are light brown and crunchy.

- Bran, oatmeal, or blueberry muffins are better options than doughnuts.

- If you are a dessert lover, plan to have dessert once a week so you don't feel deprived or unrewarded for your day-to-day efforts. Choose your moments carefully and don't overdo it. Sherbets, fruit ices, and frozen tofu desserts are all good options. You can also eat low-fat frozen yogurt once in awhile. The best dessert for you, of course, is fresh fruit in small quantities.

Beverages

- Drink six to eight glasses of water every day. Distilled water, spring water, low-sodium mineral water, and soda water are all good choices.

- Bottled water should be ozone-treated to help prevent bacterial growth. The best water is either distilled or has undergone reverse osmosis and deionization.

- As stated in the carbohydrate section, you should dilute a fourth of a glass of unsweetened juice with three-fourths of a glass of water or soda water.

- Keep your intake of caffeinated beverages to a minimum. Two cups of coffee a day should be your maximum. Drink it black with no sugar.

- Try green tea, herbal teas, or hot water and lemon as an alternative to coffee or regular tea.

- Diet drinks that contain aspartame are the most acceptable soft drinks, but don't overdo it. There is no nutritional value whatsoever in diet soft drinks; and some research calls into question the safety of aspartame, as mentioned in Step 1.

- Avoid all beverages sweetened with sugar.

- Beware of high-sodium drinks. They make your body retain sodium and water, creating a bloating effect. They also impair your body's ability to rid itself of toxins and metabolic debris.

- Tap water is always an unknown quantity. It may be wise to attach a purifier to your water tap. Reduce the amount of tap water you drink as much as possible.

- The occasional alcoholic beverage is acceptable, but moderation is the key.

- You can increase the amount of fluids you get by eating foods that have a high water content. The following foods contain more than 80 percent water: lettuce, celery, broccoli, collards, snap beans, watermelon, carrots, skim milk, radishes, raw cabbage, beets, oranges, grapefruit, and tangerines.

Appendix 4

Monthly Body Shape Assessment

Using a scale and a tape measure, enter your current weight and body shape measurements in the Month 1 column. Every four weeks, record your weight and girth measurements and enter them in the columns that follow. This tracking form will enable you to see the changes to your body shape over time. Make extra copies if you wish to record your progress beyond a year.

- Waist measurement: taken at the level of the navel
- Hip measurement: taken at the widest point around the hips and gluteal area
- Thigh measurement: taken on each leg at level just below the gluteal fold (where your buttock ends and your thigh begins)
- Calf measurement: taken at widest point around each calf
- Bicep measurement: taken at midpoint of upper arm with arm in a relaxed position hanging by the side
- Chest measurement: taken at widest point around chest (often at nipple level)

Parameter	Month 1	Month 2	Month 3	Month 4	Month 5	Month 6	Month 7	Month 8	Month 9	Month 10	Month 11	Month 12
Weight												
Waist												
Hip												
Thigh												
Calf												
Bicep												
Chest												

Appendix 5

Target Blood Levels for Optimal Health

The following blood tests will help establish the parameters against which your health and anti-aging status can be evaluated. I suggest they be included in the roster of tests administered by your physician during your annual physical exam. Note that health care plans may not cover the costs of all of these tests.

Ideal or target fasting blood results (blood drawn after a 12-hour fast) associated with anti-aging and disease prevention:

Blood Test	Target Conventional Units	Target SI Units
Glucose	Less than 90 mg/dL	Less than 5.0 mmol/L
Total Cholesterol	150-160 mg/dL	3.89-4.14 mmol/L
HDL-cholesterol	Men: above 45 mg/dL Women: above 55 mg/dL	Men: above 1.17 mmol/L Women: above 1.42 mmol/L
LDL-cholesterol	Less than 100 mg/dL	Less than 2.6 mmol/L
Triglycerides	Less than 100 mg/dL	Less than 1.13 mmol/L
Hemoglobin	135-180 G/L	13.5-18.0 g/dL
Homocysteine	Less than 1.08 mg/L	Less than 8 mumol/L
Serum Ferretin	Men: 20-300 ng/mL Women: 20-150 ng/mL	Men: 44.94-674 pmol/L Women: 44.94-337 pmol/L
Albumin	33.0-46.0 G/L	3.3-4.6 g/dL
Total Bilirubin	0.00-1.34 mg/dL	0.0-23.0 mumol/L

(Continued)

(Continued)

Blood Test	Target Conventional Units	Target SI Units
Blood Urea Nitrogen	Maximum 10-14 mg/dL	Maximum 3.57-5.0 mmol/L
Total Protein	60-82 G/L	6.0-8.2 g/dL
Creatinine	0.68-1.43 mg/dL	60-127 mumol/L
Insulin-like Growth Factor-1 (IGF-1): individuals over 40 years of age	240-275 ug/L	240-275 d/L
Vitamin D	34-48 ng/mL	85-120 nmol/L
Vitamin E	Above 1.18 mg/dL	Above 27.5 mumol/L
Vitamin C	Above 0.88 mg/dL	Above 50 mumol/L
Uric Acid (urate)	3.03-7.57 mg/dL	180-450 mumol/L
Selenium	Above 120 ug/L	n/a
Carotene	21.5-26 ug/dL	0.4-0.5 mumol/L
Prostate-specific antigen (PSA) Males Only	Less than 4 ng/mL	Less than 4 mug/L

PREFIXES DENOTING DECIMAL FACTORS

PREFIX	SYMBOL	FACTOR
mega	M	10^6
kilo	k	10^3
hecto	h	10^2
deca	da	10^1
deci	d	10^{-1}
centi	c	10^{-2}
milli	m	10^{-3}
micro	mu	10^{-6}
nano	n	10^{-9}
pico	p	10^{-12}
femto	f	10^{-15}

References:

1. Burtis CA, Ashwood ER (eds): *Tietz Textbook of Clinical Chemistry.* Philadelphia, WB Saunders, 1994.

2. Conn RB (ed): *Current Diagnosis,* 9th ed. Philadelphia, WB Saunders, 1997.

3. Hardman JG, Limbird LE, Molinoff PB, Ruddon RW (eds): *Goodman and Gilman's The Pharmacological Basis of Therapeutics,* 9th ed. New York, McGraw-Hill, 1995.

4. Henry JB (ed): *Clinical Diagnosis and Management by Laboratory Methods,* 19th ed. Philadelphia, WB Saunders, 1996.

5. Tietz NW (ed): *Clinical Guide to Laboratory Tests,* 3rd ed. Philadelphia, WB Saunders, 1995.

6. Gey KF, Moser UK, Jordan P et al. Increased risk of cardiovascular disease at suboptimal plasma concentrations of essential antioxidants: an epidemiological update with special attention to carotene and vitamin C. *Am J Clin Nutr.* 1993; 57(5 Suppl): 787S-797S.

7. Academy of Anti-Aging Research (Fellowship Program) Continuing Medical Education Series (www.a3r.org).

8. *Dr. Anderson's Antioxidant Antiaging Health Program* (Carroll & Graf Publishers) 1996: 47-48.

9. Russo MW et al. Plasma selenium levels and the risk of colorectal adenomas; *Nutrition and Cancer* 1997; 28(2):125-129.

Appendix 6

Resources

Supplementation Sources

To meet the needs of my patients and as recommendations to other health care professionals, I have formulated a number of supplement products in the course of my consulting practice. These formulations are available under the Nutra Therapeutics brand name and are fully described at www.nutra-education.com. Nutra Therapeutics can be contacted by telephone at 1-888-251-1010, should you or your health practitioner have further questions. While these products contain the exact formulations I suggest, there are other reputable manufacturers of nutritional supplements that you may wish to investigate. I have included here several cutting-edge products that I have used personally or have recommended due to their superior formulations or proven clinical efficacy.

1. Multi-Vitamin and Mineral (Nutra Therapeutics)—contains the levels of antioxidants, B-vitamins and other vitamins and minerals for anti-aging and health-promotion purposes recommended in Step 2.

2. Nature's Essential Oils (Nutra Therapeutics)—contains the amounts of essential fatty acids from borage seed oil, fish oil, and flaxseed oil for anti-aging and health-promotion purposes recommended in Step 2.

3. Body Burn—Weight Loss Supplement (Nutra Therapeutics)— contains the levels of chromium, hydroxycitric acid, and coleus forskohlii to help encourage body fat reduction as discussed in Step 4.

4. Cardio Essential (Nutra Therapeutics)—contains the levels and standard grade of coenzyme Q10 and hawthorn (as well as the flavonoid quercetin) recommended after age 40 to support heart health, brain and immune function as discussed in Step 5.

5. Immuno-Detox Prime (Nutra Therapeutics)—contains the levels and standard grade of nutrients that support the immune system and liver's detoxification enzymes after age 40 (indole-3-carbinol, milk thistle, reishi mushroom extract, astragalus) as discussed in Step 5.

6. Glucosamine Joint Formula (Nutra Therapeutics)—contains the pharmaceutical-grade glucosamine sulfate, along with MSM and other anti-inflammatory herbs, recommended after age 40 to help prevent erosion of joint cartilage and inflammation, and to help repair joint degeneration, as described in Step 5.

7. Prostate 40 Plus (Nutra Therapeutics)—contains the levels and standardized grades of natural agents recommended to help prevent and reverse prostate enlargement and support prostate health after the age of 40, as discussed in Step 5.

8. Women's Hormonal Support (Nutra Therapeutics)—contains the levels and standardized grades of black cohosh, soy extract and gamma-oryzanol recommended for the management of PMS, fibrocystic breast disease, uterine fibroids, endometriosis, menopausal symptoms and for anti-aging purposes in postmenopausal women as described in Step 5.

9. Cholestat—Cholesterol and Lipid Lowering Supplement (Nutra Therapeutics)—contains the levels and standard grades of gum guggul and policosanol recommended to help lower cholesterol and triglyceride levels, as discussed in Step 1.

10. Brain Complex (Nutra Therapeutics)—contains the levels and standard grades of nutrients recommended to support memory and cognitive function after the age of 50, as discussed in Step 5.

11. SX Primer—For Enhanced Libido and Performance (Nutra Therapeutics)—contains the levels and standard grades of nutrients recommended to support libido and sexual function for men and women over 40 years of age, as discussed in Step 5.

12. Growth Hormone Secretagogue Products:

   - PRO hGH Symbiotropin and Meditropin (Neutraceutics); learn more about these products at www.meditropin.com.

   - I also like the secretagogue product produced by Destiny Health and Wellness known as ReVie (www.destinywellness. com, 1-888- 878-9193)

13. Protein Shake—MEGAFIT Protein Blend (Destiny Health and Wellness)—contains whey and casein protein, amino acid complex, digestive enzyme complex, lecithin, and L-glycine. It is low in fat and carbohydrate calories and is sweetened with stevia, not aspartame.

   - Protein Shake—ProLab ProWhey Protein—22 grams of Whey Protein per scoop.

14. Creatine—MEGAFIT Creatine Blend (Destiny Health and Wellness)—contains creatine monohydrate to increases explosive power, along with L-glutamine, which is an anti-catabolic amino acid (helps prevent muscle breakdown during exercise and stress); 14 grams of carbohydrate and alpha-lipoic acid, which enhance uptake of creatine into muscle tissue.

   - Prolab Creatine Monohydrate Powder—a high grade, reliable source of pure creatine monohydrate.

Anti-Aging Physicians

To find a qualified physician near you who is a member of the American College for the Advancement in Medicine or the Academy of Anti-Aging Medicine, visit these websites: www.acam.org and www.worldhealth.net.

A Select Book List for Further Reading:

Here are my recommendations for additional reading on the subjects of wellness and anti-aging:

1. *Grow Young with HGH* by Dr. Ronald Klatz (HarperPerennial, 1997).
2. *Stop Aging Now* by Jean Carper (Harper Collins, 1995).
3. *The Super Anti-Oxidants* by Dr. James Balch (M. Evans and Company Inc, 1998).
4. *The Real Vitamin and Mineral Book* by Shari Lieberman (Avery Publishing Group, 1997).
5. *Fats and Oils* by Udo Erasmus (Alive Books, 1986).
6. *Cancer & Nutrition* by Dr. Charles B. Simone (Avery Publishing, 1992).
7. *Dr. Anderson's Antioxidant Anti-aging Health Program* (Carroll & Graf Publishers, 1996.

Dr. James Meschino's Website

To review the extensive list of research papers I have written, products I have formulated, or to listen to internet radio interviews I have conducted with key health authors and researchers, visit www.nutra-education.com.

Index

disease(s)
-resistant diets, 22, 31-32, 42
Crohn's, 96, 97, 236
degenerative, 2, 9, 12, 13, 64,
85, 95
peripheral vascular, 92
reducing risk of, 2, 7
vitamin-deficiency, 70
see also specific type of disease
disulfide compounds, 12
DNA
damage, 27, 65, 71, 74, 90-91,
180, 194, 217, 272
replication, 187
synthesis and repair, 90, 91

E

eggs, 33, 34, 46, 47, 57, 135,
157, 162
emotional eating, 139, 141-142
energy
from carbohydrates, 6, 7, 8, 18
from glucose, 6
requirements, 6-7
enzymes
5-alpha-reductase, 194, 202
5-lipoxygenase, 239, 240, 241
acetylcholinesterase, 248
alpha-hydroxylase, 222
antioxidant, natural, 73, 76, 87
carcinogen removal, 9
catalase, 73, 87
coenzyme Q10 (CoQ10), 79,
173-182
cyclooxygenase, 239, 240, 241

detoxification, 9, 183-185
digestive, 6, 18
estrogen synthase, 218
formation, 46
glutathione peroxidase, 73, 76,
87
liver, 6
mixed-function oxidase, 184
myrosinase, 188
quercetin, 242
superoxide dismutase, 73, 87,
187
estrogen(s)
beta-estradiol, 211
decline in, 108, 204, 205-206
endogenous, 101
estradiol, 214, 260
estriol, 214
estrone, 9-10, 11, 196, 211, 214
and flaxseed, 101-102
green tea blocking, 63
phyto-, 9, 101, 104, 188, 201,
217, 220
production, 120, 255
rise in, 194, 271
synthase enzyme, 218
exercise
-haters, 119-121, 129-130
aerobic, 109, 110-115, 116, 121,
123-128, 200
benefits, 1, 2, 64, 109, 110,
114, 120, 129
body shaping, 115, 116, 118,
119, 123, 126, 129
burning calories, 120, 122, 164

U
ultraviolet light
  see cancer (skin), eyes

V
varicose veins, 13, 22, 26
vegetables
  asparagus, 10-11
  calcium in, 49, 50
  carbohydrates in, 5, 9
  cholesterol crunchers, 25
  cruciferous, 9-10, 160, 185,
    186, 188, 199, 324
  daily intake, 20, 73
  dark-blue, 13
  dark-green leafy, 10-11, 13, 49,
    52, 86, 160, 325
  fiber in, 25, 28, 209
  iron in, 52
  juices, 10, 65
  low-glycemic, 9-12
  onions and garlic, 12, 160
  orange-yellow, 13
  potatoes, 15, 21, 57, 162, 324
  protein in, 54
  tomatoes, 10, 159, 160, 202,
    203
  Two Staple Nutrition System,
    160-161
vegetarians, 20, 32, 41, 52, 136
vitamin B2 (riboflavin), 185
vitamin B3 (niacin), 100, 185
vitamin B6, 92, 93, 94, 100
vitamin B12, 51-52, 90, 92, 93,
  190

vitamin C
  brain protection, 178
  cancer protection, 88-89, 181,
    204, 227
  daily intake, 90
  detoxification supplement, 185
  eye disease protection, 86,
    87-88
  hormone synthesis, 101
  immune system protection,
    89-90, 191
  infection, protection against,
    190
  respiratory improvement, 190
  wrinkle prevention, 88-89
vitamin D, 47, 48, 49, 77, 94,
  95, 136
  25-hydroxy, 222, 226, 228,
    230, 231
  calcitriol (1,25 dihydroxy-),
    222, 223, 226, 228, 231
  and calcium, 224-225, 227,
    228
  cancer protection, 202-203,
    204, 226-229, 230
  deficiency, 224
  from sunlight, 202-203, 223,
    229, 230
  immune system improvement,
    222
  multiple sclerosis protection,
    222, 229, 230
  osteoporosis protection, 210,
    222-225, 230
  reducing effectiveness, 223